Jenny Smith

Education
and Public Health

*Natural Partners
in Learning for Life*

ASSOCIATION FOR SUPERVISION
AND CURRICULUM DEVELOPMENT
ALEXANDRIA, VIRGINIA USA

Association for Supervision and Curriculum Development
1703 N. Beauregard St. • Alexandria, VA 22311-1714 USA
Telephone: 800-933-2723 or 703-578-9600 • Fax: 703-575-5400
Web site: http://www.ascd.org • E-mail: member@ascd.org

Project Team
Theresa C. Lewallen, *Editor*
Pamela Karwasinski, *Production Manager*
Ginny Reardon, *Project Manager*

ASCD Staff
Gene R. Carter, *Executive Director*
Diane G. Berreth, *Deputy Executive Director for Policy and Planning*
Theresa C. Lewallen, *Director, Health in Education Initiative*
Pamela Karwasinski, *Program Coordinator, Health in Education Initiative*
Gary Bloom, *Director, Design and Production Services*
Georgia McDonald, *Senior Designer*
Eric Coyle, *Production Specialist*

Support for this book was provided by a grant from The Robert Wood Johnson Foundation, Princeton, New Jersey.

All Web links in this book are correct as of the publication date below but may have become inactive or otherwise modified since that time. If you notice a deactivated or changed link, please e-mail health@ascd.org with the words "Link Update" in the subject line. In your message, please specify the Web link, the book title, and the page number on which the link appears.

Printed in the United States of America.

10s/03
ASCD Stock No.: 103380
ASCD member price: $ 5.95   nonmember price: $ 7.95

Library of Congress Cataloging-in-Publication Data
Smith, Jenny
    Education and Public Health: Natural Partners in Learning for Life/Jenny Smith
ISBN: 0-87120-826-1 (pbk.)

13 12 11 10 09 08 07 06 05 04 03   12 11 10 9 8 7 6 5 4 3 2 1

EDUCATION *and* PUBLIC HEALTH

Natural Partners in Learning for Life

◆ ◆ ◆ ◆ ◆

Introduction

Founded in 1943, the Association for Supervision and Curriculum Development (ASCD) is an international, non-partisan education association dedicated to the success of all learners. In an effort to help build a healthier student population that is ready to learn and is more knowledgeable about public health, ASCD partnered with The Robert Wood Johnson Foundation to create the Health in Education Initiative.

According to Gene Carter (2003, p. 28), ASCD Executive Director, "Our students need to be prepared to become contributing members of society, armed with the knowledge and skills to make healthy decisions and progress at solving the health issues in their lives and communities."

A fundamental mission of ASCD's Health in Education Initiative has been to encourage the development of dynamic curriculum models that promote awareness of public health among middle, junior, and high school students. The initiative awarded 10 two-year grants—$20,000 for each year—to schools or districts that partnered with community-based public health organizations to educate students about the public health field. Through this project, students identified and explored public health issues affecting their communities while also learning about careers in public health.

Education and public health are natural partners in learning. By focusing on real community health issues, students have the opportunity to develop critical thinking and problem-solving skills, which fosters their ability to make better decisions about their own health. This is particularly relevant at the middle and high school level, when youth are more susceptible to engaging in high-health-risk behaviors.

A partnership between education and public health also enhances the connection students feel toward their schools and communities. Youth learn their role in improving the health of the community by exploring current health concerns and developing authentic interventions. When students feel a strong sense of connection or belonging, they are generally more committed and they behave more responsibly. This is an important stepping-stone toward becoming responsible, contributing members of society.

In this era where many school systems and social service agencies face increasing financial strain, it is imperative that schools and public health organizations collaborate to adequately meet the needs of their communities. These partnerships can yield incredible benefits for everyone involved. In the following pages you will learn about the best practices and lessons gleaned from the experiences at schools that participated in the collaboration between ASCD and The Robert Wood Johnson Foundation.

1

Learning for Life

Nothing can more effectually contribute to the Cultivation and Improvement of a Country, the Wisdom, Riches, and Strength, Virtue and Piety, the Welfare and Happiness of a People, than a proper Education of youth.

—Benjamin Franklin (Larabee, 1961, p. 422)

Children go to school to learn fundamental skills and subjects. But the mission of education is much greater than that. Historically, the mission of schools has been to help children grow into productive, responsible adults who help make the world a better place. This is still true today. Americans feel that one of the main purposes of education is to prepare students to become responsible citizens (Rose & Gallup, 2000).

Yet many youth feel little connection to their schools and communities. They are at risk of entering adulthood lacking the commitment necessary to sustain relationships and the responsibility to participate in a democratic society (Carnegie Council on Adolescent Development, 1989). When asked about their goal in life, many students say it is simply to make money (Billig, 2000). They will soon join the ranks of young adults who show little interest in their communities or engaging in civic life (Allen, 2003; Glickman, 2003).

Although schools alone cannot be responsible for the type of citizens their students become, the school climate, curriculum, and 1 educational practices can have a lasting influence on the direction students take in their lives. With over 95 percent of youth age 5 to 17 enrolled in school (U.S. Department of Education, 2001), this institution has the greatest influence on a child's life outside of the family. Schools, therefore, play an essential role in cultivating the moral character and citizenship of their students.

The role that schools have in developing engaged citizens has been obscured by recent pressure from high-stakes testing, tight budgets, and the challenge of teaching a diverse population of students at all levels of ability. If schools want to succeed today in light of these pressures, they need to do things differently. Administrators and teachers must be innovative. They must teach differently and think about education in a new way in order to attain the goal of producing educated, responsible adults.

Schools that are effectively able to create supportive learning communities share certain influential qualities: (1) the relationships between adults and children are respectful; (2) everyone—staff, students, and parents—feels a sense of belonging; (3) students have ample opportunities for self-direction and collaboration; (4) the curriculum is challenging and engaging; and (5) the school promotes safety and community (Learning First Alliance, 2001, pp. 1–2). These schools are better able to improve academic achievement and develop the kinds of characteristics in students that lead them to become productive, responsible citizens.

Health and Education

Good health supports successful learning. Successful learning supports health. Education and health are inseparable.

—Desmond O'Byrne (2001)

Health is like a silent partner to education. The health and well-being of children are directly linked to their academic performance (Novello, Degraw, & Kleinman, 1992). In order to learn, students need to be healthy. Compared to children with physical, emotional, or mental health problems, students in good health can concentrate better in school, which facilitates academic achievement.

The relationship between health and education is reciprocal (Novello et al., 1992). Good health facilitates learning, and well-educated children are generally healthier. Through education students gain the knowledge and the skills to access information and resources for a healthy lifestyle. Educational success has been shown to contribute more to health than any other long-term intervention (Deutsch, 2000).

The sad reality is that approximately one in four children is at risk of academic failure because of physical, emotional, or social problems (Dryfoos, 1994). Most students in poor health have difficulty learning. Distracted by pain or discomfort, they are unable to concentrate on schoolwork. As a result, many act out or withdraw. These early dysfunctional coping strategies can establish lifelong patterns that set children on a downward spiral. They become disengaged from their schools and ultimately from their communities. With a limited education, they face diminished chances of making a decent living. They spin their wheels trying to make ends meet. Some become dependent on society, taxing valuable resources.

Dental problems, lead poisoning, asthma, and infectious childhood diseases caused by inadequate vaccine protection and poor prenatal care are some of the more common preventable health problems that adversely affect a student's educational development (Kinsey & Walker, 2002; Kozol, 1991; Novello et al., 1992). But physical ailments are not the only health issues plaguing students. Between 10 and 21 percent of the children in the United States have an emotional or mental health problem (U.S. Department of Health and Human Services [U.S. DHHS], 1999). Many children have no health insurance coverage (Dryfoos, 1994) or lack access to good health care, so their emotional and physical conditions often go undiagnosed and untreated.

Nationwide, many adolescents engage in behaviors such as alcohol and substance abuse, tobacco use, and sexual activity that place them at risk of serious health problems (Grunbaum et al., 2002). Studies have shown that regardless of ethnic background or social class, students who have trouble with schoolwork engage in high-health-risk behaviors (Blum, Beuhring, & Rinehart, 2000). These poor coping strategies exacerbate their situation. It's a vicious cycle for some children that only gets worse as they attempt to alleviate their untreated physical, mental, or emotional pain by turning to alcohol, marijuana, or tobacco.

How U.S. Students Fare

◆ Approximately 25 percent of all children are at risk of academic failure because of physical, emotional, or social problems, according to one estimate (Dryfoos, 1994).

◆ Almost 21 percent of the children in the United States ages 9–17 have a diagnosable mental or addictive disorder associated with at least minimum impairment (U.S. DHHS, 1999).

◆ As many as half of all youth are at moderate to high risk of drug abuse, sexually transmitted diseases, teen pregnancy, and injury or death resulting from violence or accidents (Hawkins & Catalano, 1990).

◆ Compared with students in other developed countries, middle-class whites and many Asian groups in the United States are doing reasonably well by most measures, but black and Hispanic youth experience severe health and learning inequities (Deutsch, 2000).

◆ Students who are hungry, sick, troubled, or depressed cannot function well in the classroom, no matter how good the school (Carnegie Council on Adolescent Development, 1989).

The physical, mental, and emotional obstacles to learning are greater in schools with a high proportion of low-income and poor students whose families do not have the resources for or access to adequate health care. For example, dental problems are a typical health issue affecting poor children (Kozol, 1991). Their parents cannot afford the cost of dental care and may be unaware of proper dental hygiene. The constant discomfort these students endure day after day from an impacted tooth erodes their energy and capacity to learn.

Ethnic minorities in the United States also face greater health risks than their middle-class white counterparts. According to Charles Deutsch (2000, pp. 8–9), director of the National Committee on Partnerships for Children's Health, "Adverse health and education outcomes coincide most powerfully in the persistent disparities related to race and class." Health and education are necessary complements, he believes, "if we hope to address the pervasive health impediments to learning that arise from and perpetuate disparities."

Schools Can Make a Difference

Some people feel schools cannot or should not take on health issues. Yet we know there is a direct relationship between good health and academic outcomes. Because health affects a child's ability to learn and 95 percent of the youth in the United States are enrolled in school, it is important that schools take health issues on. Fortunately many health problems can be prevented with treatment or appropriate interventions.

Rhode Island has one of the highest rates of lead poisoning in the country. "What's most frustrating," says Joseph McNamara, health and wellness coordinator for the Pawtucket School District in Rhode Island (Checkley, 2000, p. 7), "is knowing that it's totally preventable." In Pawtucket approximately one in five children tests high for lead levels when they start school. "The cost of lead poisoning—the lost potential, the neurological disorders—is too high." McNamara sees schools as critical vehicles for educating students and the public about lead poisoning.

Most serious illnesses and early mortality are the result of high-health-risk behaviors established in childhood. Six of these behaviors can be altered to prevent disease or death: poor eating habits, physical inactivity, tobacco use, drug and alcohol abuse, accidental or intentional behaviors causing injury, and sexual activity resulting in unwanted pregnancy or sexually transmitted diseases (Kolbe, 1990). Education can help prevent children from developing these behaviors.

Preventable behaviors established in childhood
◆ Poor eating habits
◆ Physical inactivity
◆ Tobacco use
◆ Alcohol and drug abuse
◆ Accidental or intentional behaviors causing injury
◆ Sexual activity resulting in unwanted pregnancy or sexually transmitted diseases

More than 80 percent of the school districts across the United States require schools to teach health education, and many have adopted the National Health Education Standards (Centers for Disease Control and Prevention, 2001). These standards, released in 1995 by the Joint Committee on National Health Education Standards, provide guidelines for teaching students to understand and obtain basic health information and services to enhance their health. Schools and districts can use the guidelines as a framework for developing their own strategies and curricula for teaching health education.

Highlights of the National Health Education Standards

The National Health Education Standards describe what students should know about health and what health education should enable them to do:

◆ Students will comprehend concepts related to health promotion and disease prevention.
◆ Students will demonstrate the ability to access valid health information and health-promoting products and services.
◆ Students will demonstrate the ability to practice health-enhancing behaviors and reduce health risks.
◆ Students will analyze the influence of culture, media, technology, and other factors on health.
◆ Students will demonstrate the ability to use interpersonal communication skills to enhance health.

◆ Students will demonstrate the ability to use goal-setting and decision-making skills to enhance health.

◆ Students will demonstrate the ability to advocate for personal, family, and community health.

(Joint Committee on National Health
Education Standards, 1995)

Although the National Health Education Standards are an important step toward healthier students, no accountability system exists to assure the effectiveness of the health education that students receive. In 2000, the Centers for Disease Control and Prevention's Division of Adolescent and School Health (CDC-DASH) conducted a study on school health policies and programs. Findings from the study revealed that although some progress has been made, health education in many schools and districts is not nearly as effective as it could be (Kolbe, Kann, & Brener, 2001).

Compared to the first CDC-DASH study conducted the year prior to the release of the National Health Education Standards, the percentage of schools that require health education increased in the elementary grades, but decreased from 27 percent in 6th grade to only 2 percent in 12th grade. Unfortunately schools provide less health education in the upper grades even though adolescents are more likely to engage in high-health-risk behavior. Required health topics are often sandwiched into classes devoted to other subjects, decreasing the time spent on the topic and the effectiveness of learning it (Kolbe et al., 2001).

The connection between health and education must be fostered if students are to succeed. The most effective health education programs are systematic, integrated, and coordinated efforts (Marx, Wooley, & Northrop, 1998). They have been shown to reduce behavior problems, increase attendance, enhance relationships, and improve student achievement. Creating an effective health education program takes no more time in the long run than dealing on a daily basis with students' health issues. Educational success depends on schools addressing their students' physical, mental, and emotional barriers to learning.

Kids are vulnerable and, if not educated, take a lot of risks. Many parents do a great job of keeping kids healthy . . . but sometimes it's just not enough, and we have to help.

—Robin Fleming, director, Cross-Cultural Education in Public Health, Seattle Public Schools (Checkley, 2000, p. 4)

2

Why Public Health?

*Health care is vital to all of us **some** of the time but public health is vital to all of us **all** of the time.*

—C. Everett Koop, MD, former U.S. Surgeon General
(Association of Schools of Public Health, 2003)

What Public Health Is and What It Is Not

Public health is a social institution many of us have heard of but would find difficult to describe. We'd likely either group public health with the medical profession or define it as the local health department. Because most of us rarely come in direct contact with public health professionals, we lack firsthand experience with this field. Yet our health is as dependent on public health as it is on medicine.

Medical personnel provide us with health care when we need it. We go to them for annual checkups and shots or to be treated for a specific illness or disease. In contrast, public health care professionals work on ways to prevent health problems that affect large segments of the population. For example, with epidemics like AIDS or severe acute respiratory syndrome (SARS), the public health profession educates society about these diseases in order to minimize occurrences.

Medical professionals work with individual patients, and public health professionals focus on the community as a whole. Medical professionals concentrate on diagnosing and treating specific ailments of individual patients; public health professionals emphasize prevention and health promotion using a variety of interventions that target the environment, public policy, and human behavior. Both medicine and public health are necessary complements in the overall health of our society.

Public Health	vs.	Medicine
Focus on population		Focus on individual
Emphasis on prevention, health promotion for the whole community		Emphasis on diagnosis and treatment, care for the whole patient
Biological sciences central, stimulated by major threats to health of populations		Biological sciences central, stimulated by need of patients
Varied interventions targeting the environment, human behavior/lifestyle and medical care		Predominant intervention is medical care
Public service ethic, tempered by concerns for the individual		Personal service ethic, conditioned by awareness of social responsibilities
Variable certification of specialists beyond professional public health degree		Uniform certification of specialists beyond professional medical degree

(Fineberg, 1990)

Public health uses a population-based approach to health. Here are some examples of how this approach works:

◆ Prevents pollution of our air and land through enforcement of regulatory controls and management of hazardous wastes;

◆ Ensures that our drinking and recreational waters are safe;

◆ Eradicates life-threatening diseases such as smallpox and polio;

◆ Controls and prevents infectious diseases and outbreaks such as measles, HIV/AIDS, tuberculosis, and the Ebola virus;

◆ Reduces death and disability due to unintentional injuries through the formulation of policies designed to protect the safety of the public, such as seat belt and worker safety laws;

◆ Facilitates community empowerment to improve mental health, reduce substance abuse, and social violence;

◆ Promotes healthy lifestyles to prevent chronic diseases such as cancer, heart disease, and obesity;

◆ Educates populations at risk to reduce sexually transmit-ted diseases, teen pregnancy, and infant mortality;

◆ Ensures access to cost-effective care; and

◆ Evaluates the effectiveness of clinical and community-based interventions.

(Association of Schools of Public Health, 2001)

Why Public Health in Education Matters

A dynamic public health curriculum in schools matters because it can accomplish several important educational goals. It teaches students about health and how to access information and health care services. It strengthens students' connection to their school and communities. It exposes students to potential careers in the public health sector. And it is also an effective vehicle for learning because public health can be integrated into the curriculum across disciplines.

The benefits of public health in education

◆ Provides an effective vehicle for learning;

◆ Teaches students about health and how it affects society and history;

◆ Strengthens the connection between students and their school or community;

◆ Encourages an interdisciplinary, integrated approach to health; and

◆ Exposes students to careers in public health.

Education and Application

Public health is a real and concrete way for middle and high school students to learn about health issues. Effective public health education includes opportunities for students to become actively involved in solving current school or community health problems. Through public health, students learn about an issue, develop a plan to address the issue, and implement interventions. For instance, in the public health approach to obesity as a school health concern, students would review data about the issue, learn about the impact of nutrition and physical activity on weight, and identify changes that can be made in the school to address obesity. A potential solution might be to replace soda machines with bottled-water machines. Students learn about good health through their effort to improve the health of others. They apply their knowledge and skills in the classroom and community, under the guidance of the instructor. Feedback is immediate and correction or reinforcement takes place in an ongoing way.

Strengthen Connections

The teenage years are normally a time of self-absorption and self-centeredness. Public health education shifts teens' focus by encouraging students to develop a sense of responsibility for others. Concentrating on the health of others strengthens students' connection to their school and community. A strong attachment to the school community and a commitment to education are critical in reducing a student's risk of drug use and delinquent behavior (Hawkins & Catalano, 1990; Resnick et al., 1997). A feeling of connectedness to school consistently leads to better health among children (Battistich & Hom, 1997; Blum & Rinehart, 1998).

An important component of any public health curriculum is service learning. ASCD's Health in Education Initiative projects used public health as the focus for a wide range of service learning opportunities across different disciplines. Service learning helps build a bond between students and their school or community and lays the foundation for becoming responsible, contributing citizens (Billig, 2000). Broadly speaking, service learning engages students in structured activities based on the needs of the school or community. It integrates the curriculum into these activities, enabling students to apply their skills and knowledge. Through service learning students develop a deeper caring for others (Billig, 2000).

Service learning, as a teaching strategy, is also a powerful way to motivate youth and build self-esteem. Studies indicate that in many cases, students who participate in high-quality service learning programs are more likely to attend class punctually, initiate questions, and complete assignments. They care more about doing their best and show greater concern toward others. Because service learning boosts self-esteem and self-efficacy, students are less likely to engage in risky behaviors (Billig, 2000).

Service learning
◆ Links to academic content and standards;
◆ Involves young people in helping to determine and meet real, defined community needs;
◆ Is reciprocal in nature, benefiting both the community and the service providers by combining a service experience with a learning experience;
◆ Can be used in any subject area as long as it is appropriate to learning goals; and
◆ Works for all ages, even young children.

Service learning is *not*
◆ An episodic volunteer program;
◆ An add-on to an existing school or college curriculum;
◆ Logging a set number of community service hours in order to graduate;
◆ Compensatory service assigned as a form of punishment by the courts or by school administrators;
◆ Only for high school or college students; or
◆ One-sided, benefiting only students or only the community.

(National Commission on Service-Learning, 2002)

Public health is an excellent vehicle for the learning process because it can easily be integrated into curricula. English classes, for example, can explore literature with health themes, math classes can analyze and plot data relating to health epidemics, and social studies classes can examine health epidemics among various cultures. Incorporating public health into these subjects facilitates the learning process and provides a variety of service learning activities.

Middle and High School
Public Health Service Learning Activities

School*	Examples of Service Learning Activities
California	Mentored and taught 10 lessons to 3rd graders about substance abuse.
Kentucky	Organized and held a one-day summit on drugs, alcohol, nutrition, and sexuality for 6th graders.
Massachusetts	Designed research and presented findings on post-9/11 hate crimes and depression among teens in a public forum with local health and city officials.
Minnesota	Educated 30 high school classes about the environmental impact of a local coal-burning power plant.
New York	Created a play for middle school students on tobacco, targeting Latino teens, as part of the advocacy efforts of the National Cancer Institute.
Pennsylvania	Created a public service announcement on carbon monoxide poisoning for local television.
Rhode Island	Created and distributed to classes, preschools, and parent support groups a nutrition guide and cookbook for combating effects of lead poisoning.
Washington	Developed and submitted recommendations for Internet articles on ethnic concerns about health care access, gangs, police, and school system issues.
Utah	Created a health-oriented newsletter distributed to the student body and faculty.

*   This list of schools, identified by the state where they reside, received Health in Education Initiative grants through ASCD to form partnerships with public health organizations in order to promote awareness of public health among middle, junior, and high school students.

Exposure to Careers

Students can gain exposure to public health careers through mentoring and internship opportunities, guest speakers, field trips, and by developing public health interventions for the school or community. Through modeling, students learn about potential career opportunities. Students of all races and ethnicities benefit from exposure to careers in public health, particularly if guest speakers and mentors have a similar ethnic background. Attracting ethnic students to careers in the health care field is also important because each ethnicity has its own nuances that are better understood by a professional with the same ethnic background.

A public health professional is involved in one or more of the following 10 essential public health services.

Ten essential public health services
- Monitoring health status to identify community health problems;
- Diagnosing and investigating health problems and health hazards in the community;
- Informing, educating, and empowering people about health issues;
- Mobilizing community partnerships to identify and solve health problems;
- Developing policies and plans that support individual and community health efforts;
- Enforcing laws and regulations that protect health and ensure safety;
- Linking people to needed personal health services and assuring the provision of health care when otherwise unavailable;
- Ensuring a competent public health and personal health care work force;
- Evaluating effectiveness, accessibility, and quality of personal and population-based health services; and
- Researching for new insights and innovative solutions to health problems.

(Public Health Functions Steering Committee, 1994)

Both public health and education strive to improve the well-being of our society. The mission of education is to create an actively engaged citizenry. The mission of public health is to create a healthy population. The education system educates individuals to improve the community. Public health promotes environmental and social change to improve the lives of individuals. Together they are natural partners in learning for life.

What Public Health Teaches

A high-quality public health education class should teach students key skills and information in three main categories: (1) general public health skills, (2) issues relating to culture with a focus on access to care, and (3) environmental change. The class must involve a well-planned service learning component if it is to be maximally effective. Instruction should also center on real and current school and community health issues.

General public health education starts with fundamental theories and models of public health in which the community is viewed as the patient. Students learn to interpret health data for their school or community to accurately understand the prevalence of disease in populations and subpopulations. Analyzing health issues helps students develop critical thinking and problem-solving skills. Interventions, developed and implemented by the students, cultivate leadership skills. Students also gain an understanding about the impact of legal and family systems on public health.

Understanding cultural issues and access-to-care issues is critical for comprehending health problems of the larger community. Family conditions and cultural values may, for example, prohibit or prevent the use of certain traditional medical practices. Language barriers may limit access to care for non-English-speaking people unable to explain their ailments or understand the medical system. Students learn about these issues through exploring their own family and cultural beliefs and that of subpopulations within the school and community.

Advocacy is also an essential component of the public health profession and an important skill for cultivating an active citizenry. A curriculum that focuses on public health issues and skills gives students opportunities to get involved in policy development or change at the school or community level. Concentrating the project's efforts in policy areas where students can be successful builds their competency and esteem. Students learn that they *do* have a voice and can initiate change that positively affects the lives of others.

When planning the public health curriculum, it is important to help students assess key public health skills they already have. The curriculum should include activities that

- ◆ Develop students' leadership skills;
- ◆ Develop critical thinking skills and problem-solving skills; and
- ◆ Expose students to the range of jobs and careers in public health, including jobs that affect public health but do not require advanced public health education, such as lead abatement or water sanitation. Consider how to replenish the field of public health and how to help more people choose public health as a career.

Essentials of a Public Health Class

1. **General public health skills**
   - ◆ Theories, models, and the language of public health.
   - ◆ Population-based approaches—the community as patient.
   - ◆ Multiple intervention approaches and the range of population impacts—students can identify which are appropriate to use in a given situation.
   - ◆ Data analysis that focuses on a specific geographical area and a particular population or subpopulation.
   - ◆ Public health systems and the impact of legal and family systems on public health—students can do an analysis of their community's system.

2. **Cultural issues and access to care**

   - ◆ Cultural beliefs and access-to-care issues for different nationalities and subpopulations. A bottom-up approach uses students from the target populations to address local community public health issues.
   - ◆ Access to family health histories to explore the population risks that increase family members' likelihood of disease (e.g., blacks—diabetes and heart disease; Caucasian women—osteoporosis).
   - ◆ Mentoring opportunities that match students with mentors of similar backgrounds.

3. **Environmental change**

   - ◆ Public policy's impact on public health—focus on what students can affect in the environment, legislature, and through increased community awareness and education.
   - ◆ Interventions that are appropriate to the public health issue and affect the environment.
   - ◆ Asset building as prevention, to reduce risky behavior and unhealthy environments.

3

Partnerships

Communities that are eager to improve the health of specific at-risk groups have found that they are more likely to be successful if they work collaboratively.

—U.S. DHHS (2000)

Key to Success: Strong Partnerships

Fifty years ago schools were smaller and student populations far more homogenous. Today many classrooms are filled at or beyond maximum capacity with economically and racially diverse students, some of whom lack English language proficiency. Schools alone cannot possibly address all the health issues of their students. They need to work with other agencies and institutions in the community concerned with the health of children. The ability to form close collaborations will ultimately improve outcomes for both health and education.

The most successful Health in Education Initiative projects involved strong, collaborative partnerships with various community groups invested in health. Some partnerships began with existing relationships; others formed new relationships. While building and sustaining partnerships requires work, they offer valuable educational opportunities to students. Partnerships with a public health agency or a university can provide professional development for staff, mentoring opportunities, public health career modeling, classroom speakers with expertise, and university interns to assist with the class. Equally important, partnerships offer the capacity to foster service learning opportunities for students.

Every partner must benefit from the collaboration in some way in order to sustain the partnership. To attract potential partners, be sure to consider how they could benefit; each may stand to benefit in different ways. Start by looking at who might already be at the school and at the school district office with an expertise in the health field or an enthusiasm for new projects. When searching for partners in the community, begin with natural allies in the health field, such as public health departments and mental health agencies.

Look for partners at colleges or universities that offer health-related programs of study. A number of undergraduate and graduate level programs require students to engage in research or community projects for credit toward their degree. Professors may also be interested in collaborating as a way to conduct research or expand outreach in public health or health education.

In the initial stages of development, bring every partner to the table to determine goals and plan the project. This helps build commitment. Be sure not to dominate the conversation or propose a fixed plan. Instead, lay out the reason a collaborative partnership with them is necessary and what you hope the partnership can accomplish. Be ambitious but realistic. Don't share any concrete ideas you've already formulated for the project until you hear from potential partners about how they can benefit from this partnership. If you tell them your project ideas up front, most likely they will view this as your project and not take ownership for it. They may provide verbal support, but not much more.

Clarify roles and take inventory of the resources each partner can bring to the project. Partners may be able to provide teaching expertise in a specific area, connections to other health organizations, professional development training, space for the class, time to organize the curriculum, materials, and financial support. Defining the roles each partner will play limits time wasted on duplicated efforts and confusion about who is responsible for each part of the project. This does not necessarily mean that the roles will be equal or outcome benefits will be the same for each partner in the collaboration. Partners typically bring different resources, play different roles, reap different benefits, and have unequal power (Deutsch, 2000).

All collaborations, even if they begin with existing relationships, demand time and attention to maintain and strengthen the partnership throughout the project. Constant communication helps prevent misunderstandings or bruised egos. Deutsch (2000) warns that while partnerships require conscientious nurturing, they also need to focus relentlessly on results to be successful. This keeps everyone's efforts concentrated on the goals of the project.

Students Teaching Other Peers (STOP)

Belmont-Redwood Shores School District, the San Mateo County Public Health Education Program, and the Department of Health Education, San Francisco State University, California

The model

Drug use among youth was a concern in the Belmont-Redwood Shores School District, which includes Ralston Middle School. The school already had an extensive partnership network in place, so garnering support was easy. Ralston Middle School partnered with the county Department of Health Services and nearby San Francisco State University to develop a public health project on drug use at the school, called Students Teaching Other Peers (STOP). Each partner agreed to provide specific resources. The school district contributed the training site and students. The county health department offered field trip visits and job shadowing opportunities. The university's Department of Health Education provided mentors for the students and transportation to the various sites (Saldivar & Tapper, 2002).

Ralston Middle School had a pre-existing District Advisory Committee with a similar agenda on school health issues. Committee members represented a diverse mix from the school community— principals, teachers, parents, counselors, and school safety officers. The STOP directors adopted this committee as an advisory committee. The committee provided valuable feedback and guidance throughout the evolution of STOP (Saldivar & Tapper, 2002).

STOP used several reliable sources to identify drug use as a problem: community epidemiological data from the county Office of Education and Department of Health Services, the Healthy Kids Survey, and literature on high-risk behavior. Project staff developed a unique approach to address the drug problem. They designed a complex, three-tiered model of university students, 8th graders, and 3rd graders. This approach was successful, in part, because of the strong partnerships and ongoing communication (Saldivar & Tapper, 2002).

The university students involved majored in education and health education. They received training on public health issues affecting the local community and careers in public health from the county Department of Health Services. They were also trained in peer education. Each received a stipend and travel expenses to Ralston Middle School. They worked on a weekly basis mentoring, training, and coaching 8th grade students on drug education and asset-building lessons that the college students had developed. Once the 8th graders completed training in health education and presentation skills, they taught 10 health education lessons to 3rd graders at several elementary schools (Saldivar & Tapper, 2002).

Highlights of this model
◆ Modeling by different tiers of students
◆ Opportunities for student advocacy
◆ Increased awareness about a community problem
◆ Flexibility by the project partners
◆ Increasing enthusiasm for the project

Challenges
Transportation to and from the schools and university was an unanticipated challenge. Because the middle school was 30 minutes from the university, fewer college students than initially anticipated could commit to the project. In addition, the distance between the middle school and elementary schools was problematic, and attempts to involve parents were unsuccessful. Fortunately one of the project leaders and the two university interns agreed to drive the students. The project partners, in constant communication, addressed these challenges and found solutions as quickly as possible, ensuring continuity and success (Saldivar & Tapper, 2002).

Most of the 8th grade students involved in this project participated as part of a class assignment. In order to provide weekly health education classes to 3rd graders, the rigorous curriculum for the 8th graders included education on drugs, training in peer education, public health job shadowing, and presentations on what they learned about public health to peers in the health education classes at their own school. It wasn't the rigor or quantity of work that posed the biggest challenge for middle school students, but rather the diverse learning needs and discipline problems in the 3rd grade classroom. The project partners immediately addressed these obstacles by providing the middle school students with additional training on classroom management. Classroom teachers provided consultation on how to work with the students with learning challenges and special needs (Saldivar & Tapper, 2002).

Outcome

Although it is unclear whether the classes added to the 3rd graders' knowledge about health or will ultimately have an impact on their behavior, of immediate importance was the positive experience the 3rd graders had. "You were so nice that you helped us" and "I hope I can be just like you" were sentiments expressed by the 3rd graders. Modeling by the 8th graders as responsible, caring individuals may have been the most significant learning for the 3rd graders (Saldivar & Tapper, 2002).

Like the younger students, the 8th graders gained immensely from the interaction with college student mentors, who treated them as responsible, respected individuals. These middle schoolers also benefited from collaborating with their peers, learning how to work together and listen to other people's opinions and ideas. Teaching the 3rd grade students about drugs and cigarette smoking expanded the 8th graders' own knowledge about these health issues. Though many of the middle school students initially participated in the project out of obligation, their overwhelming response to the experience was positive (Saldivar & Tapper, 2002).

Enthusiasm for STOP built up over time as a result of publicity and word of mouth. The school district newsletter highlighted the project, and staff made targeted presentations to the district PTA. A successful first year piqued the interest of other elementary schools in the district. The following year, the number of 3rd grade classes participating in the program expanded. Three additional classes at another elementary were added, bringing the total to five 3rd grade classes in the project (Saldivar & Tapper, 2002).

Cross-Cultural Education in Public Health

Seattle School District with Seattle and King County Public Health, Washington

Immigration in the United States is exploding. Approximately 1 in 10 Americans is born in a foreign country (U.S. Census Bureau, 2000b). Between 1990 and 2000, approximately 7 million immigrants of various ethnic backgrounds became legal residents of the United States (U.S. Census Bureau, 2001). Though the ethnic population is a minority, the U.S. Census Bureau (2000a) predicts it will increase to one-third of the population by the year 2010. According to research, immigrants have significant problems accessing health care services (Weitzman & DuPleiss, 1997).

"There are a number of factors working against immigrants. They're new [to the United States], and they may not be aware of how to access health care. If they're people of color, they also face huge risks educationally, socially, and economically," says Robin Fleming (Allen, 2002, p. 4), codirector of Cross-Cultural Education in Public Health in Seattle, Washington. Seattle, like other urban areas of the country, is home to many new immigrants.

Bringing public health education into the classroom will boost the health literacy of new immigrants while simultaneously educating them about careers in this field. Attracting ethnic minorities to the public health field is a way to help improve access to care, because ethnic professionals are better able to understand the culture and nuances of people with similar ethnicity. They are also more inclined to serve people of similar background (Drake & Lowenstein, 1998).

The model
Fleming, an elementary school nurse, initiated this project to complement her studies in community health nursing. Focusing on

immigrants and ethnic minorities, she developed a nine-week curriculum to educate students about public health issues and careers in public health. This was a more didactic model than the project in California. Initial support for Fleming's efforts came easily through partnerships developed with the Seattle School District and public health departments of Seattle and King County.

Children who view themselves as academically capable are more apt to consider a wide range of careers, including science and medicine (Bandura, Barbaranelli, Caprara, & Pastorelli, 2001). The Cross-Cultural Education curriculum promoted self-efficacy as a way to encourage academic achievement and career aspirations of immigrants. In addition to basic health education, class discussions about discrimination, assumptions, the roots of bias, and their connection to health encouraged dialogue and critical thinking. Public health speakers of various ethnic backgrounds and a job fair with high ethnic representation provided role models and information on health and careers (Fleming, 2002).

Highlights of this model
- Flexibility and integration of the curriculum
- Student self-efficacy
- Academic achievement
- Enhanced career aspirations

The flexibility of the curriculum made it accessible to a wide variety of classrooms and emphasized different skills, depending on the particular class. For example, in a literature class students identified specific health issues and wrote to health officials about their concerns. In a computer class, students linked to a cross-cultural health Web site hosted by the University of Washington's medical center. The site highlights different ethnic groups and their cultural beliefs, expectations, and practices related to health care, which can be drastically different from mainstream American medical practice. Students contributed their own ideas for articles on the Web site about health care access, gangs, police, and school system issues (Fleming, 2002).

Challenges

Because most of the students participating in the program were recent immigrants from diverse areas of the world—including Mexico, Somalia, and Vietnam—English fluency posed a particular problem. Occasionally students benefited from interpreters or assistance from peers; but more often they struggled with comprehension, particularly in English as a second language (ESL) classes, where the majority of students had been in the country for a few years or less (Fleming, 2002).

School scheduling conflicts posed another challenge to the project. Student testing, the pre-existing class curriculum, and field trips all competed for the students' time over the course of the nine-week program. These demands limited the ability to deliver the material in a timely manner, thus constraining the effectiveness of the project. These challenges could have been minimized had the public health curriculum been built into existing curricula (Fleming, 2002).

Outcome

At the end of two school years, approximately 400 students—mostly immigrants—had participated in this public health program offered at three middle schools and two high schools in the Seattle School District. Students showed an increase in public health knowledge. Some voiced the importance of learning about health to help others from their country adjust to their new life here. Others hoped to go back to their countries of origin to bring about change, particularly around issues of sanitation and water treatment. According to pre- and post-program student surveys, many of the students also expressed an increased interest in health care careers (Fleming, 2002).

This project was initiated by a single individual as part of her master's degree work. She had verbal support from the school district and access to students, but this was the extent of the school district's involvement. Rather than a collaborative effort, the project became a specialized program she brought to the schools. Similarly, the Seattle and King County public health departments provided limited support. Although they gave their seal of approval, they were not engaged in any significant way. Once the project began, lack of communication between these partners further reduced the support necessary to sustain it.

Cross-Cultural Education in Public Health was a unique project, filling a void in programs that provide ethnic minorities with public health education. However, after the grant period ended and Fleming could no longer continue her involvement, there was no one to continue the project. Had strong collaborative partnerships been cultivated from the beginning and maintained throughout the project, or had there been infrastructure support, it is possible the project could have continued.

What We Learned: Partnerships

1. **Commitment**
    - Explore collaboration versus stand-alone model to be sure you are willing to commit to a partnership.
    - Once committed, take a team approach: get input and involvement from all partners. Every voice needs to be heard.

2. **Potential partners**
    - Look for who is already there. At the school or district level: superintendent, district health program coordinator, principal, school nurse, school health councils, science and social studies teachers, subject area experts, any other energetic open-minded teachers who like to take on new challenges, school-to-career staff, guidance counselors, parents of students, and any school-community committees. In the community: public health agencies, mental health agencies, health departments, organizations providing services to youth, and local colleges or universities.
    - Consider what every partner has to gain from the collaboration. Partners can provide access to resources previously unavailable or untapped by schools.

◆ Get to know the reality of all the players involved: district, school, teachers, students, public health agency, and university. What are their needs and limitations? What do they hope to achieve from the collaboration?

3. Build and maintain

◆ Set clear goals. Be ambitious but realistic. Don't try to accomplish too much at once, particularly at the beginning, when you are trying to figure out how to make the project succeed.

◆ Combine the most important public health and education skills, knowledge, language, and issues. Although education and public health are somewhat related in their intent, they have different ways of carrying out their tasks. In a true partnership it is important to know the differences and to integrate them.

◆ Clarify roles. All partners may not have an equal role, and that's okay.

◆ Be sure all partners are committed. Keep in mind that commitment can be expressed in a variety of ways. But if a partner fails to follow through, check in to find out what's going on.

◆ Communicate frequently throughout the project. Keep each other abreast of everything you do—this helps prevent misunderstanding, hurt feelings, and missed opportunities. Be sure to include parents in some of the communication to build outside support for the project.

◆ All relationships require time and attention, and partnerships are no exception.

4

Champions and the Infrastructure

Key to Success:
Multiple Champions and Infrastructure Support

Infrastructure support

For any new project to thrive, a supportive infrastructure must be in place. Take time to honestly examine how open your school culture is to new ideas, particularly new ideas that rely on the involvement of outside agencies and institutions. Does your school support the notion that it's okay to receive input and help from others? Does your school support teamwork among teachers? An open, collaborative environment is best for this kind of project. Or at the very least there must be a genuine willingness to be open-minded and cooperative. Problems will arise from the start without genuine support for the collaboration from administrators or teachers.

Overcoming obstacles

With increasing pressure on school schedules and demands for time in the curriculum, many teachers and administrators are concerned about the time required to begin something new. Public health education does not need to be an add-on that requires more time from everyone involved. Use the existing infrastructure; don't start from scratch. Appropriate school and community committees can address the need for a project like this, brainstorm ideas, and formulate a plan of action. Existing advisory committees can oversee the project and provide feedback. Summer workshops, continuing education classes, or inservice training sessions are useful arenas in which to develop a public health curriculum. Curriculum choices may depend on which educators are interested in presenting the material, or public health education may be integrated into existing curricula, refocusing and reframing lesson plans.

Keep your expectations and needs realistic. Use what you have in order to accomplish what you can. Budget cuts may limit access to financial resources; however, exclusive reliance on outside monetary resources to accomplish your project will lead to its demise once the funding runs dry. Use any available finances frugally and be sure to budget for necessary student incentives like snacks, awards, or stipends. Work with existing projects and resources. This is where partnerships can be particularly useful, because they can provide things you may not be able to supply.

Staff turnover, common in schools and community public health agencies, occurred in many of the Health in Education Initiative projects. Changes in staffing, scheduling, and policy can create enormous disruptions. In order for the project to survive during upheavals, it is critical to have strong champions in each of the partner organizations. Solid leadership is important to maintaining the enthusiasm and functioning of any project. Transitions did not have a negative impact on the project overall when it had multiple champions and infrastructure support.

Obstacles
◆ Hectic work schedules
◆ Starting from scratch
◆ Budget cuts
◆ Staff turnover
◆ Schedule conflicts
◆ Class interruptions
◆ Insufficient time to cover all the material

Coping strategies
◆ Keep expectations and needs realistic.
◆ Work with existing resources.

- ◆ Piggyback on existing infrastructure, curricula, and projects.
- ◆ Realistically assess challenges.
- ◆ Develop strong champions in each partner organization.

Multiple champions

Cultivate champions in each partner organization. This means obtaining more than their verbal support for the project. Get them involved in a way that serves their own needs so they are invested in the continuity of the project. Don't be afraid to come right out and ask them what they need and how this project can help them accomplish it. Be prepared, however, to adjust your own needs in order to accommodate theirs. Remember, another organization's needs could add to the project and strengthen it in a way you had not initially anticipated.

Involve all partners in planning and development. Since the roles of each partner are different and not necessarily equal, once the project begins some of the partners typically become less engaged. It is important to the success of the project to maintain a high level of commitment from these less-involved partners, even though they are no longer essential to the daily operation of the project. You need to be able to turn to your partners for assistance in the *likely* event of staff turnover or unforeseen challenges. Keep the project on their radar screen through meetings and ongoing communication. Foster ongoing enthusiasm among the partners by talking up the accomplishments of the program and promoting successes through local events or in the media.

Acknowledge the potential for project staff turnover and determine in advance who will step in at each partner organization should this occur. Involve these backup people in some way, especially at training sessions. Send them written communication about the project so they begin to develop an interest in and an allegiance to it. Realize, however, that if the school principal leaves, the groundwork will need to be laid again to gain the support of the successor, even if there are other advocates at the school. The same applies to other organizations when there are top management staff changes.

Ways to cultivate multiple champions
◆ Get key people involved from each partner organization.
◆ Involve all partners in planning and development.
◆ Keep the project on the radar screen of key people.
◆ Promote successes.
◆ Cultivate backup people at each partner organization.

College Exploratory Program in Public Health

William Howard Taft High School, Bronx-Lebanon Hospital, and Hunter College, New York

Approximately 165 students at William Howard Taft High School in the South Bronx participate in the school's Academy of Health. Since 1990, this four-year academic enrichment program has provided career exploration in the health care field through mentoring, internships, job readiness training, and specialized classes in health education. In order to offer students a class in public health—which could better prepare them academically by developing skills in critical thinking, epidemiological research, computing, and public speaking—the school needed assistance from the community (Roberts, Cordero, & Pichardo, 2002).

The partnerships: old and new
Taft High School's Academy of Health and nearby Bronx-Lebanon Hospital already had an established working relationship. The school formed a new partnership with Hunter College of the City University of New York for this project. Each of the partners had something different to gain from the collaboration, and their roles in the project varied.

An assistant professor in the college's Urban Public Health Program became an ally in this project. She developed and taught the curriculum for the high school's College Exploratory Program in Public Health class, with input from the Academy of Health coordinator. The class was held on the university campus. Faculty and staff from another area of the college, the School of Health Sciences, facilitated class workshops and provided use of their research and teaching facilities. The Nutrition and Food Science program at the college, for example, gave a workshop to the high school students using state-of-the-art equipment to measure body mass index and prepared a nutritionally balanced meal in their food lab (Roberts, Cordero, & Pichardo, 2002).

College student interns in the Urban Public Health Program assisted in the development, implementation, and evaluation of the class. They also served as mentors to the high school students. During the first year of the class, the project staff included three interns—two graduate students and one undergraduate. The second year, staff increased to seven graduate student interns. College interns received academic credit for their participation in the project as well as a small stipend (Roberts, Cordero, & Pichardo, 2002).

Access to the college was a boon for the high school. According to Lynn Roberts (personal communication, May 7, 2003), assistant professor in the college's Urban Public Health program, the socioeconomic status of South Bronx, where Taft High School is located, rates as one of the lowest in the country. Many of the students have learning challenges, and the school is considered one of the most troubled in New York City. For students who have never been on a college campus before, taking a class at a college can be an exciting experience that opens the door to future possibilities.

The model

The College Exploratory Program in Public Health class took place on Saturdays. Although teenagers generally are not keen on attending school on Saturday, holding the class at Hunter College provided the draw. Students had the opportunity to use the college library and laboratory while also learning about campus life. The course provided them with a stimulating and challenging academic experience.

Roberts made a presentation to promote the class at a special assembly for Academy of Health students. A number of students enthusiastic about learning something new signed up; however, several others registered for different reasons. Participants received a small stipend to cover lunch and transportation to the college. The first year, 15 students registered and 10 completed the course. The following year, 20 students registered and 15 saw it through to the end. The students who did not complete the class mostly dropped out because of personal or family problems, though a few did not meet attendance requirements and were not allowed to continue (Roberts, Cordero, & Pichardo, 2002).

The small class size proved to be beneficial in a number of ways. Project staff found it easier to monitor students and follow through with accountability. The smaller class allowed the teachers and mentors to give students individual attention. Although many of the students did not follow through with homework assignments, they stayed well beyond classtime once they were engaged in more interesting, hands-on projects with the university mentors (Roberts, Cordero, & Pichardo, 2002).

"When you have kids like these coming from troubled homes, they liked that we were interested in them," said Roberts (personal communication, May 7, 2003). The students thrived under the attention, the responsibility, and the high expectations the college had for them.

During the course's first year, students selected their public health projects. However, the second year the director decided that the students should participate in an opportunity to collaborate with the National Cancer Institute (NCI) on a tobacco-use prevention campaign targeting Latino youth. The students did not like losing the freedom of choosing their own topic, but soon found they could put more effort into developing their interventions because they did not have to start from scratch with materials, resources, and data (Roberts, Cordero, & Pichardo, 2002).

Multiple champions

An unusual partnership developed the second year that gave students the chance to be involved in a health education campaign for NCI. A college student in the public health program who also worked with the Cancer Information Service at NCI received a fellowship to develop a tobacco-use prevention campaign with input from Latino adolescents from New York City. She approached the college professor who codirected the high school College Exploratory Program in Public Health class. The class decided to make tobacco their focus, and student teams developed strategies to implement a public health education campaign. This authentic student engagement experience provided students with the opportunity to "learn by doing" (Roberts, Cordero, & Pichardo, 2002).

Another partnership developed because of the high school students' initiative. Students on one of the intervention teams created a play called "It's Your Choice, You Pick, Don't Smoke!" for younger children. Without prompting from their mentors, they approached their former middle school principal about presenting their play at his school. The principal arranged a presentation of their play to the entire 5th grade. Although the middle school participated less than other partners, its involvement contributed significantly to a successful academic experience for the Academy of Health students (Roberts, Cordero, & Pichardo, 2002).

The college interns were also important champions. Although they were primarily drawn to the College Exploratory Program to fulfill internship requirements, their participation added immensely to its success. Only two of the interns had experience working with high school students, yet their support and commitment to these adolescents went well beyond what was expected of them. It was not unusual for them to meet outside of class to assist the high school students with research projects and other public health assignments. With their experience and skills, these college students were excellent role models (Roberts, Cordero, & Pichardo, 2002).

The College Exploratory Program had infrastructure support because it easily fit into the high school's successful Academy of Health. Even so, when the school's project director retired, he took the extra step to ensure he had a successor. By establishing support for the project from the new Academy of Health coordinator, turnover had minimal impact. During the new school coordinator's transition and orientation, the project leaders at Hunter College and Bronx-Lebanon Hospital maintained the continuity of the project.

Highlights of this model
◆ Good fit with existing infrastructure at the school
◆ Willingness to expand beyond the school campus and structure
◆ Access to a university
◆ High expectations and accountability of students
◆ Individual attention because of small class size

◆ New partners added throughout the process
◆ Continuity through staff turnover maintained by multiple champions

Challenges

School restructuring by the superintendent's office proved to be a great obstacle the second year. During the transition, communication between the school staff and the other partners decreased, resulting in missed opportunities for collaboration. For example, the Hunter College team did not learn that the high school health clinic was offering a series of smoking cessation workshops until the students in the public health class began conducting a Knowledge, Attitude, and Behavior survey on tobacco use among the student body. With better coordination, it might have been possible for the public health students to assist the school health clinic staff in workshop planning and recruitment based on the survey data the students gathered (Roberts, Cordero, & Pichardo, 2002).

Despite the breakdown in communication with the school during the second year, the class remained intact and continued along a productive course. The school restructuring did not threaten the survival of the class because there was solid infrastructure support for it. The new coordinator of the Academy of Health bought into the class, the Bronx-Lebanon hospital gave its support and input, and there were multiple champions at the university, headed by the professor in the Urban Public Health program (Roberts, Cordero, & Pichardo, 2002).

Outcome

At the end of the year, the high school students presented their public health projects at a culminating event on the college campus with a keynote speaker. The 100-member audience included college faculty and interns, schoolteachers, administrators, and family members. This event put more pressure on the students than if they had only presented their projects to their classmates. As a result, the students concluded this experience feeling a great sense of pride and accomplishment (Roberts, Cordero, & Pichardo, 2002).

Healthy Me + Healthy You = Healthy Schools and Healthy Neighborhoods

Thurgood Marshall Elementary School and the LaSalle Neighborhood Nursing Center, Pennsylvania

Thurgood Marshall Elementary is a Title 1 school for children in kindergarten through 8th grade. It is located in a distressed inner-city neighborhood of Philadelphia. Living in an environmentally and economically impoverished community, these children are at high risk for physical, mental, and emotional health issues. Lead poisoning, asthma, and infectious childhood diseases because of inadequate vaccine protection are some of the more common preventable health problems (Kinsey & Walker, 2002). This population stands to benefit greatly from collaborative efforts between health and education.

The model

LaSalle Neighborhood Nursing Center at La Salle University joined together with the Philadelphia School District to create an education and community service project in public health for 7th and 8th graders at Thurgood Marshall Elementary. With the principal's support, a number of teachers and staff got involved—the school nurse, the technology teacher, the art teacher, the kindergarten teacher, and the computer skills teacher. The LaSalle Nursing Center brought nursing and dietary students into the classroom and provided field trips to the university (Kinsey & Walker, 2002).

The public health curriculum initially fit into the pre-existing health instruction time slot. Input from the school nurse and a review of adolescent health data and local environmental issues determined the health topics. Using a combination of role-play, art, video, lecture, research, and field trips, students learned about nutrition, exercise, childhood lead poisoning, dental health, asthma, and drugs (Kinsey & Walker, 2002).

Highlights of this model
◆ Targeted high risk community
◆ Flexible curriculum

◆ Catalyst for public health outreach efforts
◆ Fostered community awareness

Unexpected benefits

The project was the catalyst for a number of good public health outreach efforts. A school health survey was conducted using the School Health Index developed by the CDC-DASH. The survey assessed the effectiveness of the school's current health policies and promotional efforts. Student representatives worked with school staff, university student nurses, and the public health nurse to analyze the data and provide a report to the principal for future planning. Students also conducted an environmental and economic health assessment of the neighborhood. They identified relevant public health issues and resources available in the community (Kinsey & Walker, 2002).

During the summer the project continued with a camp. Students participating in the summer program were excited to visit the university and learn about environmental health issues. The curriculum focused exclusively on the topic of carbon monoxide poisoning, a pertinent community health issue as a neighborhood family had died the previous winter when they left their car running in a closed garage. As an intervention project, students created a public service announcement for television that still airs today on a university station (Kinsey & Walker, 2002).

During the second year, the project provided the only health education to 8th graders at the elementary school. Because of low test scores, the district eliminated health education from the curriculum. The LaSalle Nursing Center staff worked closely with the school to provide health education to the 8th graders through the project (Kinsey & Walker, 2002).

Challenges

Most of the students attending Thurgood Marshall live in poverty and, as a result, have considerable mental, emotional, and physical barriers to learning. A number of the students performed well below grade level and could not read or write. Others had behavior problems. Lacking direct classroom experience, the nurses and nursing students from LaSalle struggled with class instruction and classroom management problems. School stability, support, and resources were needed to help this project succeed (Kinsey & Walker, 2002).

Challenges facing this model
◆ Financial instability
◆ Uncommitted district and school staff
◆ Lack of ownership or pride in the project by some partners
◆ Emotional and physical obstacles to learning
◆ Difficulty with classroom management

Unfortunately the school district, troubled by a financial crisis, underwent drastic changes that reverberated throughout the school.

Even though the principal at Thurgood Marshall originally backed the project, the district changes demanded much more of his time and attention. Many of the teachers initially involved in the project left the school, and eventually the principal also resigned. There was no ownership or understanding about the project among the new staff as the school scrambled to readjust to all the transitions (Kinsey & Walker, 2002).

Health education was eliminated from the curriculum; therefore, the project had to find a new home. By shifting the focus to environmental health issues, the project could fit into the science curriculum. Many of the same topics could be covered—asthma, lead poisoning, air pollution—by concentrating on how the environment affects health. However, changes in teaching assignments and schedules no longer made it feasible to offer the course to 7th graders, reducing the number of participants to two 8th grade classes (Kinsey & Walker, 2002).

Although the curriculum found a new home in science, other districtwide and staffing changes disrupted the overall success of the project in the second year. When the school district reorganized and terminated the position of the school liaison, who had been the project champion in the district, the level of support at the school was difficult to maintain. Without multiple champions and infrastructure support, a project like this cannot survive the kind of upheaval and turnover experienced at this school (Kinsey & Walker, 2002).

What We Learned:
Champions and the Infrastructure

1. The infrastructure

◆ Be sure there is support at the school and district. Is your school project-friendly and open to new ideas? Is it a school that supports teamwork? Is the district supportive of the project?

◆ Look for what's already in place. Use existing infrastructures to brainstorm and develop ideas and curriculum. Tap into school-community committees, summer workshops, and school inservice professional development sessions. Incorporate existing data such as community health assessment, Youth Risk Behavior Survey, and state health data. Piggyback on current projects and work with existing curricula. Don't reinvent the wheel.

◆ Identify community resources. Find out who can offer what and use what you have in order to do what you can.

◆ Set up an advisory council to oversee the project and to provide support and ongoing feedback.

◆ Provide professional development. Be sure to include backup teachers in training sessions.

2. Multiple champions

◆ Cultivate champions in each partner organization. If you can bring more than one advocate into the project from each organization, that is even better.

◆ Take steps to maintain the involvement of each partner organization through ongoing communication, meetings, and efforts to publicize the accomplishments of the program.

3. Common challenges

◆ Multiple champions require—on everyone's part—willingness to compromise.

◆ If the school principal leaves, you must lay the groundwork again to gain support from school administration.

◆ Staffing changes are likely to occur. Acknowledge the
potential for staff turnover and determine in advance
who would step in at each partner organization should
this occur. Be sure to involve these backup people in
orientations, training sessions, and communication about
the project.

5

Single Focus

Key to Success: Select a Single Focus

Students are more likely to become health literate when the curriculum focuses on a single public health issue with a strong service learning component. Concentrating on one topic allows for much greater depth in learning and instruction. The impact is more lasting. Students learn skills they can use to access services and resources pertaining to any health issue to make better decisions about their own health and well-being.

If the class is focused on one topic, everyone can share resources and materials. It is also easier to coordinate service learning activities, thereby providing students with opportunities to practice intervention and advocacy skills in a real context. Through authentic learning experiences, students gain a deeper understanding of public health.

The argument in favor of including a number of fundamental health issues in the curriculum is understandable, because many communities experience multiple public health concerns—nutrition, physical activity, tobacco use, drugs, alcohol, and sexually transmitted diseases, for example. Although these topics are all equally important, ASCD found that the most successful projects focused on a single issue. Moreover, they concentrated on an issue relevant to the school or local community. For instance, in Rhode Island where lead poisoning is nearly twice the national rate, this became the single focus for the public health curriculum to the exclusion of all other community health topics.

In ASCD's experience, classroom instruction suffered at schools that studied more than one or two public health topics. The volume of information required for each issue spread the class focus too thin. Learning was superficial and students didn't gain a true understanding of public health. Teachers and project coordinators also found the workload far more time-consuming and cumbersome when they needed to learn about and teach multiple public health issues.

Benefits of selecting a single focus
◆ Greater depth in instruction and learning
◆ Sharing of resources and materials
◆ Easier coordination of service learning
◆ Ease of integration across the curriculum
◆ Targeting of impact on the community

Integration across the curriculum
A single focus facilitates integration across the curriculum and across the school environment. While some projects created an entirely new public health education class, others incorporated public health into the existing curriculum. Integration of public health education can make learning a deeper and richer experience for students as they explore different aspects of a health issue through various subjects. A math class, for example, may analyze and chart the health data for the school. An English class might write articles for the local newspaper to raise awareness about community health issues and changes that could support healthy behaviors.

Health education is commonly taught in isolation without either integration into the curriculum or opportunities for students to practice their new skills in the school environment. Although this method is much easier than reworking the curriculum and creating a school environment where students can try out skills acquired in class, it is less effective. Students need to learn about healthy choices, but they also need to be supported in their ability to make those choices. What good is talking about physical activity if there is no physical education class at the school? What good is learning about good nutrition if the available food isn't healthy?

Incorporating public health into the existing curriculum requires staff to rethink the subjects they are teaching and create new lesson plans. This demands extra effort up front, but it is far more effective than tacking public health on to another subject. Once an integrated curriculum has been developed, it also requires less time and fewer resources than creating and maintaining an entirely separate public health class.

Choosing an issue

With a single focus, staff can predetermine the issue or allow the class to choose. For greater success, the public health issue should be immediately relevant to the school or community. When selecting a topic, be sure to consult several epidemiological sources. Find out what health data already exist for your school or community at the local health department, mental health department, or public health office. If class time is tight, predetermining the issue might make more sense. However, if there is time, experience shows that students will have greater enthusiasm and a more authentic experience if they are given the opportunity to analyze the data and choose the public health issue themselves.

> **Two ways to select a single topic**
> ◆ Predetermined by staff
> > **Pros:** Uses available resources and materials; more class time available for service learning.
> > **Cons:** Less buy-in from students; less student responsibility.
> ◆ Selected by students
> > **Pros:** Strong student support; opportunity for students to analyze data.
> > **Cons:** Time-consuming.

Children learn better when the subject matter is real and of interest to them (Curtis, 2002). Choosing a topic relevant to the school or community provides a genuine context for learning. Additionally, when service learning activities are focused on a real issue, students are given the chance to affect their environment in a way that helps others. This empowering experience teaches that they can have an impact on their community in a positive way. It helps to cultivate their identity as responsible, contributing citizens.

Lead Smarts

Pawtucket School District, the Rhode Island Youth Guidance Center, Rhode Island Department of Health, and Memorial Hospital, Rhode Island

NOTE: A more detailed description of the student engagement activities is included in Chapter 6: Student Engagement in the Community.

A critical issue: lead poisoning

As paint chips and peels off the walls in the historic buildings dotting Rhode Island's skyline, children are exposed to its harmful effect. The rate of lead poisoning in Rhode Island is among the highest in the country, affecting 8.1 percent of the children under 6 years of age (Rhode Island Department of Health, 2002). Compared to the national rate, twice as many children in Rhode Island have lead levels in their blood that exceed the standard of concern set by the CDC. Further, the rate of poisoning mirrors racial disparities. One in five black children in Rhode Island is identified with lead poisoning, owing primarily to the large proportion of ethnic groups living in urban areas where lead poisoning rates are highest. Lead paint is the most common source of poisoning, although lead is also found in contaminated soil, dust, and water.

The sale of lead paint was prohibited in 1978 (Rhode Island Kids Count, 2003). Little was done, however, to remove the lead paint that already covered the walls of homes. The damage wreaked from lead toxicity can be permanent and fatal, resulting in seizures and death (Wooler & Herman, 2002). Even low levels of poisoning can be debilitating for children, causing nervous system and kidney damage, stunted growth, and hearing problems. Signs of lead poisoning in students include behavior problems, hyperactivity, learning disabilities, and decreased intelligence (Rhode Island Department of Health, 2002). Lead poisoning in adults—although less common than in children—can lead to high blood pressure, nerve disorders, memory and concentration problems, muscle and joint pain, and fertility problems (Wooler & Herman, 2002).

The good news is that lead poisoning is completely preventable by properly removing lead paint from homes and monitoring lead levels in children's blood. This is a public health issue where knowledge is the key to prevention. Therefore, it is critically important to get the word out to the community. Schools can play a key role.

Natural allies
Pawtucket, an aging industrial city in Rhode Island, is home to a growing population of new immigrants (Wooler & Herman, 2002). Many Latino and Cape Verdean arrivals are unaware of the health threat on the walls of their old homes. In 2003, an estimated 16 percent of the children entering kindergarten in the Pawtucket School District had a history of lead poisoning (Rhode Island Kids Count, 2002). This rate is even higher than their peers statewide.

When the Pawtucket School District joined forces with Rhode Island Youth Guidance Center, there was no question that lead poisoning would be the sole focus. Its relevance to the community made it a natural choice, and educating students about the dangers of lead was a surefire way to alert and inform those most vulnerable to this threat. By focusing on lead poisoning to teach students about public health, this project put into practice an essential public health intervention strategy: health promotion and education of the target population.

The movement to deal with lead poisoning was well under way at the Department of Health and Rhode Island Housing. These agencies were natural allies and became long-lasting partners. The Childhood Lead Action Project, concentrating on this issue at the public policy level, became another important and active partner. With outreach into the neighborhoods, the partners were eager to get involved in the classroom and welcomed students as interns. The school was able to ride a wave that was already happening in the community by selecting this topic (Wooler & Herman, 2002).

The model

The team developed a basic curriculum to introduce issues about lead poisoning that could be used in various subjects and classes, using guest speakers from the community agencies. Targeting middle and high school students, the curriculum covered lead poisoning facts, demographics, information on how it occurs, prevention and interventions, community resources, laws and regulations, and jobs in the field of public health relating to lead poisoning prevention and remediation. Opportunities for students to participate in school-to-career and project-based learning activities were also organized.

The initial goal of the project—dubbed *Lead Smarts*—was to establish a knowledge base by educating as many students as possible in a wide variety of classrooms. At the two Pawtucket high schools, the curriculum was integrated across subjects in a variety of classes: family and consumer sciences, child development, ESL, parenting classes for pregnant teens, school-to-career, and special education classes. In some of the subjects it initially took a slight shift in thinking to work lead poisoning into the curriculum; in others it was a natural fit. For instance, ESL teachers are always looking for good, new material to teach English language skills, so focusing on a community issue turned out to be tailor-made for this class.

At the middle school level, the Lead Smarts curriculum was taught in five classes. The final assignment required each student to create a brochure focusing on some aspect of the lead issue. Many of these ethnically diverse students designed brochures in their native language. By the year's end, approximately 500 students received lead poisoning education.

Highlights of this model
◆ Natural allies in the community
◆ Single focus
◆ Clear goals
◆ Strong outreach component
◆ Integrated curriculum across subjects
◆ Student-initiated service learning projects

◆ Public recognition
◆ Media attention

Revising the model

The project directors used the first year to sow seeds in a variety of settings using a broad-based approach. Once the groundwork was laid and community relationships solidified, the project assessment clarified what needed to be revised. In year two, the emphasis shifted to project-based and community service learning opportunities for the students in the high schools. With a core of teachers on board, the project directors could move to the next level of implementation and work directly with public health professionals to get students involved in raising awareness of lead poisoning in the community.

Evolution of this model

◆ Added project-based and service learning opportunities.
◆ Recruited more teachers.
◆ Added new classes.
◆ Increased involvement of teachers and students fostered buy-in.
◆ Heightened awareness in the community.

In the second year, the project staff actively recruited more teachers to participate in the Lead Smarts project and integrated lead poisoning into their curricula. Science classes such as chemistry, physiology, and environmental science easily incorporated lead education into their courses. Teachers determined the depth of education they would provide on lead awareness in conjunction with required student-initiated community service learning projects. Actively involving the teachers and students increased their engagement.

Challenges

In spite of regular communication between the agencies and staff, school politics was an ongoing challenge. Some teachers found it difficult to fit the lead curriculum into their subject or class because of the bureaucratic constraints imposed on them. Others, however, found ways to make the lead curriculum work. Staff had varying skills of figuring out their own roadmap within the imposed limitations.

Outcome

Diligent planning, flexibility, hard work, and dedication contributed to the success of this project. Along with a dozen teachers, approximately 200 students participated the second year. A single focus on lead poisoning fostered strong service learning activities. Nearly 75 percent of the youth reported that they helped educate others about lead poisoning through creative and varied service learning projects. Students wrote a play about lead and a nutritional guide to help minimize the effects of lead in the body. They created videos, a Web site, PowerPoint® presentations, a coloring book, and a lesson plan on lead education for younger children. They designed posters and pamphlets on lead awareness in Spanish, Portuguese, French, Russian, Polish, and Cape Verdean Creole. Various projects were showcased at the Department of Health, the Pawtucket Visitors Center, and at the 2002 Department of Health Lead Excellence Awards in Rhode Island.

It took a lot of effort and energy to build relationships and develop a curriculum to fit each class, but focusing on one issue that already had momentum in the community proved extremely beneficial. Allies came naturally and easily, eager to build and sustain partnerships to further their own objectives. Student-initiated community service learning activities gained recognition and drew media attention. With such strong community support, the project will continue in the years to come.

Community Health Awareness Through Teens (CHAT)

Grand Rapids High School and the Itasca County Resource Center, Minnesota

Grand Rapids High School sits in a remote town in northern Minnesota. This rural community, with a population of 43,000, is spread out across the land. The dying steel and coal industry have taken a toll on the economy—the per capita income had fallen to the lower third in Minnesota when the Community Health Awareness Through Teens (CHAT) project started (Elhard & Lavalier, 2002). Grand Rapids High School students experienced higher-than-average rates of teen pregnancy, substance abuse, and domestic violence.

The model

The Grand Rapids High School and the Itasca Public Health Department discovered they had mutually dependent needs. The school wanted to engage students in project learning activities that strengthened their connection to the community to build resiliency and improve their health. The health department needed youth involvement on a number of committees and projects. Although the school and health department had occasionally called on each other for isolated events, through CHAT they formed a formal partnership to meet their common goal of educating students about public health (Elhard & Lavalier, 2002).

The two partners developed a curriculum for a Public Health and Community Issues class offered at the high school. Five public health issues affecting children were central to the course: fetal alcohol syndrome, child and adolescent growth and development, environmental health, violence prevention, and tobacco-use prevention. These issues were preselected by the partners based exclusively on the local Community Health Plan (Elhard & Lavalier, 2002).

Through a variety of guest speakers, class discussions, research, and surveys, students learned about the public health issues. For class assignments and intervention projects, students could choose to investigate topics of personal interest to them or relevant to the community, provided it related to one of the five issues. The students found that making a choice was not easy. They heard presentations from nearly 25 experts in the community, which pulled their attention in different directions (Elhard & Lavalier, 2002).

With 55 to 60 students in the class—many with learning challenges—the teachers found it difficult to keep students focused on intervention projects. "By the time these kids are juniors and seniors, they are trained to fill in the blanks and turn in their worksheets," explained Dan Elhard, the class instructor, "so it's tough to get them to focus." According to Elhard, this year one-third of the students in the course have special education needs and 80–90 percent are performing in the bottom half of their class.

In an effort to foster the students' sense of the role and responsibility of citizens for the health and well-being of their community, the teachers added a community service component to the class. The students had to look for ways to get involved in building the health of the community. They were required to spend a total of 50 hours during the school year at an agency that addressed one of the five public health issues. This experience exposed the students to organizations and to socially conscious adults concerned about the welfare of others. The students were surprisingly enthusiastic about volunteering in the community. For youth, this kind of exposure is an important component of lifelong learning (Elhard & Lavalier, 2002).

Challenges

Alterations in available resources threatened this project early on. Budget cuts at the school reduced the number of teachers involved in the Public Health and Community Issues class from four to two after the first year. Simultaneously, tight finances and staffing changes at the Public Health Department severely limited its involvement, creating a schism in the partnership. According to Elhard, "The time for meaningful planning was seriously lacking and led to minimal sharing of ideas between public health and teaching staff." These limitations resulted in a more teacher-driven and prescribed course than initially planned.

As originally designed, the course covered numerous public health issues, which affected the depth of the course. Two dozen guest speakers urging students to develop projects related to their particular area of expertise further scattered the energy of the class. With so many issues, disjointed community representation, and no student involvement in selecting the issues, the student intervention projects lacked meaningful connection to the community (Elhard & Lavalier, 2002).

Obstacles
◆ Large class size
◆ Focus spread too thin

- ◆ Scattered energy
- ◆ Lack of up-front student involvement
- ◆ Disjointed community representation
- ◆ No meaningful connection to the community

Coping strategies
- ◆ Flexibility
- ◆ Shift to single focus
- ◆ Stronger service component

Selecting a single focus

When the town became embroiled in a controversy regarding a proposed coal-burning power plant, the students decided to take on this issue. In doing so, they became engaged in an authentic public health experience. "It felt more real to the kids because it was a hot topic at that moment and it blew up in the community," said Elhard (personal communication, May 6, 2003).

The class concentrated exclusively on this one topic, learning as much as they could about the impact of a coal-burning power plant on the well-being of the community. They invited guest speakers from all sides of the issue—power plant representatives and their main opponents—two doctors from the medical community, and the local public health agency. Each day, students read and discussed articles from the local paper about the topic. Once they felt they understood the issue in depth, the students decided to educate their peers about what was happening in the community. To accomplish this, they made presentations to 30 classes at the high school (Elhard & Lavalier, 2002).

Outcome

By focusing all their attention on one topic, the students experienced public health at the grassroots level. They learned how to assess all sides of an issue to make good decisions to improve health. They took responsibility for educating others. From this experience they also developed skills they can use to explore other health issues.

Because the topic the students chose was an environmental health issue immediately relevant to their town, they were able to get involved and advocate for the health of their community. Their efforts were highly regarded, and students from the class were asked to represent the high school on the Community Power Plant Advisory Committee (Elhard & Lavalier, 2002).

This kind of genuine affirmation not only built the self-esteem of these youth but also fostered their connection to the community in a way that no class, guest presentation, or field trip could accomplish. The rewards these students experienced by getting involved in this authentic public health issue and working alongside public health professionals will have a lasting impact as they grow into adults. Participating in real issues, taking responsibility for others, having their voices heard and respected—this is what turns youth into productive, contributing members of society.

What We Learned:
Single Focus

1. Focus
- ◆ A single topic can be covered in greater depth. Instruction provides more opportunities for students to gain a true understanding of public health.
- ◆ It's easier to coordinate service learning activities for a single topic. Service learning is an important component to public health, and it offers students a more authentic learning experience.
- ◆ Teachers and project coordinators find the workload more manageable.
- ◆ A single issue can more easily be integrated into the existing curriculum in a variety of subjects.
- ◆ A single topic helps students become health literate. They will be able to apply their skills to access resources and services to make better decisions about their health.

2. Selecting a focus
- ◆ The topic can be predetermined by the school or public health agency, or it can be chosen by the students. Consider the pros and cons of who makes the choice.

When students choose the focus they have greater ownership, and it provides them an opportunity to analyze
community health data and use it in the decision-
making process.

◆ Choose an issue relevant to the school or local community in order to participate in community problem
solving. Don't pick something that might never occur in
your community. Analyze several sources of health data
pertaining to the school or community to be certain it is
a topic of relevance.

◆ Select an issue that is culturally relevant to the students.

◆ Consider the following when selecting a focus: Is it a
compelling issue? Is it potentially resolvable? Is a large
segment of the community affected? Does it fit well with
different courses or can it strengthen the curriculum? If
you answer "yes" to all or most of these questions, then
your focus is a good choice.

The Samples and Tools section of this book includes a tool to
help you select and prioritize your focus.

6

Student Engagement in the Community

Community service learning projects are potentially wonderful "textbooks." They involve complex problems, real-life contexts, and exposure to people who possess wide expertise and resources not found in schools.

—James Toole and Pamela Toole (1995, p. 99)

Key to Success: Service Learning

In schools with the most effective public health models, students had the opportunity to apply their skills and knowledge in a real-world context. The best outcomes occurred when students initiated their own interventions in their school or community. When learning is connected to real life, as it is in effective service learning projects, students are more committed and motivated (Curtis, 2002). The capacity for learning is far greater.

Service learning provides opportunities for authentic student engagement in the community. Effective service learning fulfills a genuine community need while also maintaining a connection to academic content. In service learning projects for public health, students get involved in creating interventions to deal with real public health issues affecting the school or community. Service learning is an excellent way for students to have a true experience of public health and learn about careers in this field.

Volunteering, like service learning, enables students to make a positive contribution to the community. However, volunteering does not engage students in the same way that service learning does (Allen, 2003; Glickman, 2003). Volunteers typically perform a task (e.g., feeding the homeless, making gifts for shut-in people, fund raising); service learning students are engaged in resolving problems. In service learning they examine data, think critically, use communication skills, interact with others, confront diversity, and develop an acceptable solution. As volunteers, students may feel good about contributing, but they generally do not experience a wide range of educational opportunities. They do not learn and grow in the same way they can through service learning.

Essential elements of effective service learning

- Engages students in service work that challenges and stretches them cognitively and developmentally.
- Requires the application of concepts, content, and skill from the academic disciplines and involves students in the construction of their own knowledge.
- Engages students in service projects that have clear goals, meet genuine needs in the school or community, and have significant consequences for themselves and others.
- Maximizes student voice in selecting, designing, implementing, and evaluating the service project.
- Prepares students for all aspects of their service work. This includes an understanding of their role, the skills and information required to perform the tasks, safety precautions, and knowledge about and sensitivity to the people with whom they will be working.
- Fulfills curricular objectives through student reflection using a variety of methods that encourage critical thinking. Reflection is done before, during, and after service work.
- Values diversity as demonstrated by its participants, its practice, and its outcomes.
- Promotes communication and interaction with the community and encourages partnerships and collaborations.

◆ Acknowledges, celebrates, and further validates students' service work.

◆ Uses assessment as a way to enhance student learning and to document and evaluate how well students have met content and skill standards.

◆ Employs evaluation of the service effort and its outcomes through formative and summative methods.

(National Service-Learning Cooperative, 1998)

The degree of implementation and effectiveness of service learning varied among the projects featured in this book. They all required students to develop public health projects. However, at some schools students did not apply interventions in the school or community; they simply presented their projects to their classmates. Although these students gained public health research skills, their projects did not constitute service learning. Students who made presentations did not have the experience of connecting their efforts to school or community improvements.

Collaborative partnerships with community agencies and institutions are critical if students are to perform interventions in the community in any meaningful way. Failure to build or maintain these partnerships made it more difficult for several of the Health in Education Initiative projects to provide students with service learning experiences. Students participating in those projects did not get the chance to truly engage in the community.

The students

For service learning to be successful, students' abilities and limitations must be considered. This is particularly important when offering a public health class that is open to all students or if the curriculum is integrated into a variety of classrooms. For example, Lead Smarts included ESL students, students with special needs, and advanced placement native speakers. The service learning projects were designed to reflect the different strengths and abilities of the students. Ideally, students should also have mentors whose backgrounds match their own.

Because most teenagers live in the moment and may be accustomed to short-term class assignments and immediate feedback, student engagement activities may pose a challenge. Be sure to clarify expectations up front. Some youth require close monitoring and follow-up. One teacher voiced concern that his students might not be capable of acting responsibly in the community; so instead, he had the students design their intervention projects for the school population.

Engaging low-performing students in service learning can be extremely beneficial. It creates a positive connection between adolescents and their community (Wooler & Herman, 2002). Lower-performing students are less likely to leave the community to attend college; they are inclined to stick around and become the future citizens of the town (D. Elhard, personal communication, May 6, 2003). If they continue their community involvement into adulthood, the community also greatly benefits.

Because we now know that everyone learns in a different way, authentic student engagement in the community offers an alternative learning experience. It might excite hard-to-reach students as well as deepen the learning for others. Although it is important that service learning be rigorous, it is equally important that students succeed in their intervention efforts.

Benefits of student engagement
◆ Alternative learning experience
◆ Involvement in the school and community
◆ Opportunity for real-world learning experience
◆ Motivation for students
◆ Increased capacity for learning
◆ Greater commitment

Evaluation and grading
Some teachers quite understandably shy away from service learning because it can be difficult to evaluate student progress. Others choose to give credit rather than a grade. As you would for any educational component, consider what students should learn or be able to do through their service learning experience. Collaborate with public health professionals or professors to develop rubrics that include demonstrations of knowledge about how public health is carried out. To measure student learning, use a variety of

methods—portfolios, reflective writing, time sheets and rating sheets, summaries by mentors or supervisors, or tangible products the students create (Witmer & Anderson, 1994).

Student reflections are an important part of service learning (Toole & Toole, 1995). They cultivate creative and critical thinking skills. Reflections can take many forms: group discussions, journal entries, short stories, speeches, drawings, slide shows, videos, and even cartoons. Prior to beginning service learning projects, reflections prepare students for the experience. During service learning, reflections give them the chance to consider their experience and ask questions, share observations, and solve problems. Afterward, reflections examine the impact of the service learning project: students can assess their intervention and evaluate what they learned in order to gain meaning from the experience and guidance for the future.

The Samples and Tools section includes suggested service learning reflection activities.

Rewards and incentives

The most successful Health in Education Initiative projects also included concrete incentives. Awards, credentials, and articles in local newspapers recognized the merits of the students' work outside of the school environment. When student engagement is authentic, incentives are often authentic. Feeling valued by the adult world bolsters self-esteem. Simultaneously, public recognition spreads the word about the project and garners community support for it while increasing the students' pride in their participation.

Since teenagers can be self-absorbed, service learning shifts their attention outward. Service learning focuses students on the health issues of the community. Through positive community service experiences, students learn the personal satisfaction that goes beyond monetary reward. As they develop a sense of responsibility for other people, the bond they feel toward their school and community strengthens, affecting academic outcomes (Billig, 2000). They become better students and better citizens as they learn the role they have in improving their community.

Considerations of service learning

◆ Strong partnerships with community agencies and institutions

◆ Realistic expectations

◆ Students strengths matched with service learning activities

◆ Mentors whose backgrounds are similar to the students

◆ Incentives

◆ Evaluation rubrics and reflections

◆ Recognition within and outside of the school environment

Lead Smarts

Pawtucket School District, the Rhode Island Youth Guidance Center, Rhode Island Department of Health, and Memorial Hospital, Rhode Island

NOTE: A more detailed description on the background of this project and why lead poisoning was selected is described in Chapter 5: Single Focus.

A significant risk factor present in many communities like Pawtucket—with a large influx of immigrants and many low-performing schools—is the alienation youth feel from where they live, according to Bob Wooler, executive director of the Rhode Island Youth Guidance Center, one of the partnering organizations in the Lead Smarts project. Many among the large population of recent immigrants feel unwelcome, and many ethnic groups and natives feel displaced. Their children don't perceive the city as a good place to live or a place to make their future (Wooler & Herman, 2002).

Most of Pawtucket's schools are low performing, with the majority of the children falling below national standards in language arts and math. Nearly a quarter of the students, ages 3 to 21, are enrolled in special education. High school graduation rates are among the lowest in the state. In 2001 only 63 percent of the seniors graduated, compared with 81 percent statewide (Rhode Island Kids Count, 2002). Lead Smarts showed that in spite of difficult circumstances, great success is possible through strong student engagement.

Service learning activities foster a connection between students and their schools and communities—replacing alienation with resiliency and promise. Students who are engaged in their community in a positive way learn about its strengths, building a sense of hope about their home. Helping to address the immediate health concerns of the community through this kind of hands-on learning also boosts student achievement. Research suggests that people become more intelligent through learning to solve problems and create products valued by society (Allen, Hogan, & Steinberg, 1998).

The model

To address the serious problem of lead poisoning among the children in Pawtucket, this school district and its partners initiated a broad-based lead awareness education campaign. Five hundred middle and high school students were taught a curriculum in lead poisoning. Once the foundation had been laid, during the second year students at the high school level initiated community service learning projects (Wooler & Herman, 2002).

A school-to-career class wrote a play about a parent's experience with lead poisoning and presented it at neighborhood elementary schools. Nutrition classes wrote a nutritional guide and cookbook with recipes full of important nutrients that help prevent lead poisoning. The book was distributed to elementary classes, preschools, early start programs, and parent support groups. Students in a media class learned how to design PowerPoint presentations illustrating the critical points of lead poisoning. In an ESL class, students learned English by interviewing each other about lead poisoning on videotape and created pamphlets and posters in their native languages. During Lead Awareness month, the Department of Health and the Pawtucket Visitors Center displayed the students' projects (Wooler & Herman, 2002).

Challenges

In spite of the engaging nature of these hands-on activities, the greatest challenge Lead Smarts staff and teachers faced was follow-through with student intervention projects. Working on time-consuming projects and making a long-term commitment to a community organization were new experiences for students accustomed to tests and brief assignments. Immediate and ongoing incentives—from snacks to stipends—helped motivate them. Although some students did not completely fulfill their commitments, those who did gained new skills and reaped personal rewards (Wooler & Herman, 2002).

Real-world incentives

One of the project partners, Rhode Island Housing, provided an exceptional real-world incentive. The education and training coordinator at the office offered to teach an eight-hour class to students on lead-safe home repair. Students who took the class and also passed the associated exam received an official certificate that allowed them to get a Lead Safe Remodeler/Renovator License. A high school industrial arts teacher, a champion of the project, enrolled all 50 of his students and followed up to be sure they attended. Nearly 20 additional students from other high school and GED classes also participated (Wooler & Herman, 2002).

All 65 students who participated in the Lead Safe Remodeler/Renovator class received certificates of completion. Twelve of them sat for the exam, receiving financial assistance from Lead Smarts to pay for the test fee. All 12 successfully passed and received a Remodeler/Renovator License. One student, who previously saw himself as a failure, got a perfect score on the exam and ran around the room with his arms up in triumph! The following year, 27 students took the Lead Safe Remodeler/Renovator class and 24 students sat for the exam. Of these, 21 students passed and were licensed. These licenses opened the doors to job opportunities for some students (Wooler & Herman, 2002).

In collaboration with Lead Smarts, Rhode Island's Department of Health, Rhode Island Housing, and the Childhood Lead Action Project created four student internship positions during the second year. To apply, students completed a lengthy application, submitted a teacher recommendation, and were interviewed by their prospective on-site mentor. The student interns worked at these agencies after school. Each intern received a $500 stipend once they completed 80 hours working at their internship site (Wooler & Herman, 2002).

A senior who interned with the Childhood Lead Action Project received training to conduct presentations on preventing lead poisoning through specific home-cleaning methods, good nutrition, and regular screening. During the course of his internship he made presentations to approximately 170 people, including children, in a variety of community venues. "It's been a learning experience," he said. "At first I didn't know there were so many kids and so many victims of lead poisoning. I just hope that by working with the community at places like the Childhood Lead Action Project, people can be made more aware and it can be stopped before it happens to others" (Wooler & Herman, 2002, p. 8).

Examples of real-world incentives
◆ Professional licensure
◆ Internship positions
◆ Stipends

Unexpected rewards
Through service learning projects and internships, Pawtucket's high school students got involved in genuine public health interventions around lead poisoning. Some gained valuable work experience to add to their resumes and college applications. The project staff worked closely with those who were unable to fulfill their assignments, keeping the experience positive to foster a favorable connection between these students and their community (Wooler & Herman, 2002).

Targeting at-risk teens, Lead Smarts' community service learning component of the project was a powerful experience for both the youths and adults. As one Pawtucket teacher said, it provided an "opportunity for the students to get involved with their community, the opportunity for me to see them as emerging change agents for a good result in the community, [and] also their opportunity to become self-confident about their ability to make a difference" (Wooler & Herman, 2002, p. 15).

Many of the students showcased their projects at Rhode Island's 2002 Department of Health Lead Excellence Awards, honoring efforts to build lead awareness. Some were even involved in the awards ceremony: Students from a high school science class made a presentation they had developed on lead awareness and two ESL students gave a brief speech advocating for greater support of immigrants and government enforcement of lead regulations. The project staff noted that it was an accomplishment for these students to speak in front of an audience and to have their voices heard by the community. The experience created a positive link in the chain that connected them to their city (Wooler & Herman, 2002).

Examples of unexpected rewards
◆ Valuable work experience for college resumes
◆ Increased self-confidence
◆ Opportunities to be valued and recognized by the adult community

Future Shock: Practicum in Public Health Research

Cambridge Public Schools, Health of the City, and the Cambridge Department of Public Health, Massachusetts

NOTE: This project is described in additional detail in Chapter 8: Administrative Support.

Cambridge Rindge and Latin School, with nearly 2,000 high school students, sits near the heart of an urban center just across the river from Boston. Like any inner city zone, Cambridge has poverty and crime. Yet this is juxtaposed with the wealth and intellect drawn to the university at the hub—Harvard. Reflecting the city's population, Cambridge Rindge and Latin School is a mix of poverty and wealth, with 40 percent of the students on free or reduced lunch (E. Grady, personal communication, May 15, 2003). It is also racially diverse: 40 percent of the students are Caucasian, 30 percent are black, and the remainder are a mix of ethnicities.

The model
When teachers from the school collaborated with Harvard University to develop a curriculum, they created a rigorous public health course targeting the more advanced juniors and seniors. The course examined historical events through the lens of public health

in all its aspects. Student-initiated research projects also addressed ethical considerations and legal issues of public health. Although students did not have to complete prerequisites to take the class, the course included statistics necessary for understanding public health data and integral to the development of the students' research projects. Because of this math component, students considered Future Shock a difficult class, and only those interested in the challenge enrolled (Grady, 2002).

The original design of the course called for a team of four teachers from different disciplines, which allowed for collaboration across subjects and a manageable distribution of the workload. The four teachers could give each student adequate support in pursing topics self-selected for their research projects. Future Shock attracted a high caliber of students, motivated and capable of working independently. Allowing freedom of choice gave the students more responsibility and pride in what they produced (Grady, 2002).

Student input was invited throughout the process of developing the research projects. Once they understood the basic concepts of public health, students used the Internet and print media to begin looking for a topic. Students also relied on the biannual Teen Student Health survey to examine data on adolescent health issues and formulate their research questions. They assessed their own learning using rubrics and peer evaluation (Grady, 2002).

Highlights of this model
◆ Collaboration across subjects
◆ Manageable distribution of workload
◆ Motivated students
◆ Historical perspective of public health
◆ In-depth analysis of ethical and legal considerations
◆ Student-initiated research projects
◆ Assessment and peer evaluation

Intervention projects seek to affect behavior, and research-based projects aim to understand and quantify behavior. The events of September 11, 2001, triggered public health research projects from several students. One investigated the rate of hate crimes in the school following the attacks. Another student researched post-9/11 depression in the school population. A third student took the topic of depression a step further to find out if a sample of depressed students were prescribed medication as their initial treatment or if other therapeutic measures were taken (Grady, 2002).

At the end of the semester, the class presented their research findings in a large public forum. This invitation-only event drew a large crowd of school and district administrators, teachers, students, parents, and members of the large umbrella health organization in the city. One of Future Shock's goals was to have the Cambridge Alliance of Health use students' findings to inform their decisions and outreach efforts. The forum was a mechanism for sharing information with the alliance (Grady, 2002).

Unlike a classroom presentation to their peers, this public forum exponentially raised the caliber of students' experience. Presenting their research findings to the larger community exposed students to an authentic and critical facet of public health. It validated that their work was of interest to people who make community public health decisions (Grady, 2002).

Challenges

After the first year, financial constraints reduced the staffing from four teachers to one. Selecting a single topic for all the students' research projects would have made the workload more manageable for one teacher, but the project directors opted not to do this. Instead, the curriculum was slightly modified to provide more time for the students to work on their research projects (Grady, 2002).

Outcome

The rigor of this class and the level of responsibility given to the students to conduct their own research made Future Shock extremely successful. The research process challenged students and provided an avenue for authentic student learning. Like true public health research, their projects had to include an abstract, introduction, materials and methods, data and results, analysis and discussion, a final conclusion with recommendations, and a bibliography. Assessment of student proficiency included benchmarks on data analysis, principles of statistics, sampling methods, and research design.

Through class assignments, students acquired valuable research and communication skills they can apply to any topic. They also learned about the social and historical impact of public health and ethical and legal considerations of research. These are important learning experiences for students as they become active citizens who vote, make recommendations at their jobs, and consider their own health decisions.

Research is an important element of public health. It is the necessary first step. This course lacks a true intervention component, which is the next step in public health. Given the motivation and research skill of these students, a service learning component could add significantly to student learning and the impact of the data on the community.

What We Learned:
Student Engagement

1. **The importance of student engagement in the community**
   - It provides a real context for applying knowledge and skills. The capacity for learning is greater when the teaching relates to real life.
   - It builds student interest and commitment because it requires active participation.
   - It provides an alternative teaching method that adds depth to the class and subject matter.
   - It fosters the connection students feel to their school and community.
   - It offers students an authentic experience of public health.
   - It spreads the word and garners political support for the project.
   - Students develop a sense of their role in making their community better through public health interventions; they learn to be better citizens.

2. **The students**
   - Decide if there will be selection parameters for the class or if it will be open to all students. How will the class have rigor and high expectations for all students regardless of their abilities? How will the curriculum and service learning be structured for students at different levels of ability or in different classes? How will the size of the class affect the service learning?
   - Know your students' abilities and limitations. Plan for immediate and ongoing incentives to motivate students.
   - Be aware of your students' cultural needs. Choose service learning activities relevant to your student population, and select mentors that match students' backgrounds.
   - Clarify academic demands—attendance, participation, and so forth. Explain the connection between public health and the students' other classwork or courses and the connection to their community.
   - Create service learning projects that are rigorous for students but will also lead to success.

3. **Different types of rewards and incentives**
   - Snacks can entice students to attend a class or event.
   - Participation can fulfill school/district/state service learning requirements.
   - Provide recognition at school or, better yet, by a community group.
   - Solicit recognition in the local media.
   - Access to a university campus is a unique experience for some kids and makes them feel older and more responsible.
   - Award a certificate from the state legislature with a picture of the group at the state capitol building.
   - Provide some sort of certification that will assist with employment.

4. Common challenges

◆ Lack of strong, collaborative partnerships with community agencies and institutions makes it difficult to create service learning experiences in public health.

◆ Evaluating and grading service learning can be a challenge. Develop rubrics and use a variety of methods to evaluate student learning.

◆ Some students require close monitoring with service learning activities. Follow up, follow up, follow up. Remember that these students have the most to gain from a favorable experience.

7

Assessment and Review

Key to Success: Ongoing Assessment and Review

What works

Ongoing assessment and review provides valuable feedback about what is working and what is not. Feedback can come from a variety of sources. Since this public health project is for the benefit of the students, getting feedback from them is critical. Feedback can also come from other teachers, student interns, and project partners. The feedback can be anecdotal or written assessments addressing specific questions. Although assessments are time-consuming, they are less time-consuming than dealing with unaddressed problems. When ongoing assessment is a part of the original plan and all the partners use the feedback, the project is strengthened.

Sources of feedback
◆ Students in the course
◆ Instructors teaching the curriculum
◆ Project partners
◆ University interns

Projects that included ongoing assessment and an overall review at predetermined intervals were better able to make necessary changes to improve the project. Projects that did not include opportunities to evaluate or were inflexible found themselves off track when something unexpected occurred. It is inevitable that challenges will arise when implementing a novel curriculum involving a new approach to community collaboration. Building in regular assessments will help identify problems early on that could derail the project.

Egos are bound to get involved in any cooperative venture. Admittedly it's difficult not to take feedback personally when some aspect of the project you are invested in is not working. A good way to prevent these occurrences from derailing a project is to keep the focus on what is best for the students and to rely on available data from assessments. Then make necessary changes to the project accordingly. By concentrating on what the data indicate and the students' best interests, there is less chance someone will take feedback personally.

Flexibility

Good project management skills include flexibility and a willingness to work around challenges or to find a new way to carry out a project. The most successful projects had directors with these skills. Assessments and reviews are a waste of time if the project leaders are inflexible.

In a school environment where unforeseen schedule changes are common or staff turnover can occur, flexibility is important. Be ready to switch gears on short notice or have an alternative plan— *Plan B*—ready. Common glitches include last-minute assemblies, field trips, or tests that conflict with scheduled classtime. Regular communication with administrators and project staff can help minimize class interruptions and provide advance notice of unavoidable schedule changes. Set priorities and improve organization so time is not wasted.

Losing staff to budget cuts, retirements, or resignations can be a difficult challenge. Prepare for staffing changes by establishing a leadership succession in case key individuals leave, and train backup staff who can easily step in.

Challenges
◆ Losing staff to budget cuts, retirements, or resignations
◆ Last-minute assemblies that cut into classtime

◆ Field trips that take students out of the class

◆ Testing that interferes with scheduled classtime

Coping strategies

◆ Flexibility

◆ Daily communication with administrators and project staff

◆ A backup plan

◆ Established priorities

◆ Improved organization

◆ Backup staff

◆ A leadership succession

◆ Focus on what is working

Highlight successes

A final note of caution: With any assessment or feedback, it is important to look for successes. Evaluations that focus exclusively on what is *not* working can be discouraging. Too much bad news might lead to defeat. "Part of the problem with evaluation is that you keep the limelight on things that don't work," says Julie Gast, a project partner from Utah State University. "You have to show what's working, too." This helps maintain enthusiasm for the project and may point to potential solutions for future problems (J. Gast, personal communication, May 7, 2003).

Planned Approach to Healthier Schools (PATHS)

Skyview High School and North Cache 8-9 Center, Utah Department of Health, and Utah State University, Utah

The PATHS project in rural Utah grew from a collaboration among professors in the Health, Physical Education, and Recreation Department at Utah State University, the Utah Health Department, and two schools: Skyview High School and North Cache 8-9 Center, a junior high. This project emphasized a remarkable level of organization and structure that ultimately contributed to its overall success. The staff's plan of action laid out a detailed schedule for curriculum development and review, opportunities for feedback from teachers and administrators, regularly planned assessments of the projects, and board meetings (Gast & Lounsbery, 2002).

Development

PATHS staff formed two distinct boards early in the project to create an organizational structure and facilitate communication among the partners. The advisory board, which directed the project and laid out the plan of action, consisted of two teachers from the university, the principals from each school, and a staff member from the health department. The curriculum board, responsible for creating the curriculum and evaluating the project, was made up of university professors, university student interns, and schoolteachers (Gast & Lounsbery, 2002).

The project directors recruited six teachers to integrate the curriculum into their subjects: biology, sociology, speech, English, and physical education. These teachers sat on the curriculum board. During the first year, the board met weekly to create the curriculum before bringing it into the classrooms. Board members developed assessment tools, created a plan to pilot the curriculum, and scheduled opportunities for feedback from students, teachers, administrators, and the local health department (Gast & Lounsbery, 2002).

Physical activity and nutrition, topics preselected by the health department, were the public health focus. This rural community had seen a rise in obesity among youth (J. Gast, personal communication, May 7, 2003), mirroring the national trend. Through educating students about physical activity and nutrition and exposing them to models from the community health profession, PATHS hoped its students would become community health educators for their schools. This approach was aimed at empowering the students and teachers with the tools they would need to make appropriate personal health decisions and to catalyze changes in the school environment that would support increased physical activity and improved nutrition.

Highlights of this model
- Broad collaboration
- An advisory board and a curriculum board

◆ A curriculum integrated into other subjects
◆ A high level of organization
◆ Detailed schedule for curriculum development and review
◆ Regularly planned project assessments
◆ Opportunities for feedback from students, interns, teachers, and administrators

Implementation

At the beginning of the second year, the curriculum was ready for implementation. At each school the teachers combined classes in a common room to team teach the public health curriculum on a designated day each week. Interns from the university's health education program assisted in the classroom and mentored the students. PATHS students learned about the relationship of good health to physical activity and nutrition. They collected data on physical activity and nutrition at their school and compared it to state and national data. Using these data, they planned public health intervention projects for their school (Gast & Lounsbery, 2002).

Feedback

Assessment and feedback are part of the university protocol. This component proved invaluable to the success of the project. The teachers, student interns, and health department staff kept journals to reflect on the merits and challenges of every class. Student feedback came from focus groups and a survey completed at the end of the semester. The curriculum board met regularly to evaluate the program based on all these sources of feedback.

Assessment tools
◆ Reflection journals
◆ Written evaluations
◆ Surveys
◆ Focus groups
◆ Board meetings

First-semester feedback and assessments made it clear that a number of challenges needed to be addressed before PATHS could continue. Students from some classes expressed frustration because they did not understand how the public health information fit in with their regular course (e.g., biology, English, speech, sociology). They did not comprehend the health promotion process or its role in public health. When they began to develop their intervention strategies, the students wasted a lot of time brainstorming impossible and inappropriate interventions (Gast & Lounsbery, 2002).

Assessments also revealed that although a lot of time had been spent developing the curriculum, little attention had been paid to the strengths and limitations of the student population. This omission created challenges in the classroom. Students did not complete assignments and seemed to lack interest in and motivation for participation in the project. The PATHS directors spent the second semester reviewing and addressing the problems revealed through the assessments and feedback (Gast & Lounsbery, 2002).

Assessment-based retooling

Back at the drawing board, the partners addressed the needs of the students and the shortcomings of the curriculum. A new course syllabus, to be handed out the first day of class, spelled out objectives and expectations. The partners abandoned the team-teaching approach because it posed problems with curriculum integration and complicated the class schedule. Instead, university interns and health department staff taught the public health segment of the class and made a deliberate effort to clarify the connection between the class subject matter and physical activity. For the first three class meetings, the curriculum was modified to standardize instruction on physical activity, nutrition, data, and health promotion. Students were also given a list of predetermined interventions to choose from so they could hit the ground running (Gast & Lounsbery, 2002).

The board created new incentives and accountability measures to motivate students. Students earned points for completed assignments, lessons, and implementation efforts; after reaching a certain point level they were rewarded with T-shirts, boxer shorts, water bottles, or pens that carried the PATHS logo. These incentive items had value for the students and proved to be good motivators.

A reflection assignment at the end of class gave students the opportunity to write down their thoughts and concerns and gave instructors the chance to address potential problems in a timely manner (Gast & Lounsbery, 2002).

Strategies used to strengthen the project
◆ Clarified objectives and expectations
◆ Explained relationship of public health information to the subject
◆ Standardized instruction in multiple classes
◆ Predetermined student intervention projects
◆ Created incentives and accountability measures
◆ Developed daily reflection assignments

Outcome
Modifications to PATHS made it far more successful. Student motivation improved and students were better able to design and implement appropriate schoolwide interventions. They created a health-oriented newsletter distributed to the student body and faculty. The students publicized *No TV Week* and drew more than 200 pledges from families. After they surveyed magazines for tobacco and alcohol advertisements, the students wrote letters to magazine publishers requesting that they stop accepting tobacco and alcohol advertisements (Gast & Lounsbery, 2002).

Students took pre- and post-tests to evaluate the overall impact of the PATHS project on the students' attitudes and behaviors related to physical activity and nutrition. Results showed that at the high school, the girls became more active and developed a better attitude toward physical activity. Teachers observed that students had higher self-esteem and were more willing to interact across peer social boundaries after participating in PATHS. The project directors and school staff attribute this change to the group work and leadership responsibilities the students had (Gast & Lounsbery, 2002).

The assessment also revealed that parts of the project were ineffective. There was no change at either school regarding attitudes about nutrition, indicating the need for future modifications to the curriculum to make it more effective (Gast & Lounsbery, 2002).

Although this project targeted the student population, it also had an impact on school staff. The faculty and staff at both schools, after seeing what the students were doing, jumped on the bandwagon and started their own wellness programs. Word about the project also extended to the state level. One of the university professors involved in the project received an invitation from a member of the state legislature to testify before a subcommittee proposing a bill to increase the amount of hours for physical education and to limit access to vending machines in schools (J. Gast, personal communication, May 7, 2003). The subcommittee was interested in learning about ways to improve the health of school children through projects like PATHS. The project also received national recognition when one of the principals received a Healthy School Hero Award at the National Healthy Kids Summit for his support of the project.

Although it can be difficult to measure the long-term impact of the students' public health efforts, the project champions did an excellent job evaluating and tracking the effects of this project. Ongoing feedback enabled them to address challenges as they arose. Pre- and post-assessments indicated that the curriculum had an impact on students' self-esteem and attitudes toward physical fitness. These assessments also pointed out where revisions needed to be made to the curriculum so it could be more effective. In addition, the project had an unanticipated positive effect on the staff at the schools and attracted attention at the state and national levels.

Mountaineer Public Health Pipeline

Ritchie County Schools, the Ritchie County Primary Care Association, and the Department of Medicine at West Virginia University, West Virginia

Located in a rural area in the northwest corner of West Virginia, Ritchie County is surrounded by an abundance of natural beauty but lacks essential social resources. When the Mountaineer Public Health Pipeline project began, over 20 percent of the population lived *below* the poverty level, and the unemployment rate was 13.4 percent. Compared to the family income levels of all 55 counties in

West Virginia, Ritchie County was near the bottom—in 45th place. The median family income was $20,584, and many families lacked medical insurance (Campbell, Thompkins, & Westfall, 2002).

This remote region was troubled by serious health issues and inadequate access to health care. A small community with slightly more than 10,000 residents, Ritchie County ranked highest in the state for cancer rates and third for infant mortality. Chronic illness and disability were common. With only three part-time physicians, two of whom covered other clinics in different regions, the medical needs of this county were sorely underserved. The demand for competent public health professionals and health care workers was great (Campbell, Thompkins, & Westfall, 2002).

Examples of regional health challenges
◆ Inadequate access to health care
◆ No health insurance
◆ Insufficient family income
◆ High rates of cancer
◆ High rates of infant mortality
◆ Chronic illness and disability

The model

Less than half of the student population in the Ritchie County schools is college bound (Campbell, Thompkins, & Westfall, 2002). The rest stay in the community and enter the work force during or immediately following high school. The school system, in partnership with the West Virginia Bureau for Public Health and the West Virginia University Health Sciences Center, hoped to spark the students' interest in public health issues and get them into the pipeline to pursue public health careers. The project partners designed a special course for high school students that fit easily into an existing School-to-Work program, in which one of the six tracks is health careers. The pronounced issues affecting the community provided a tangible opportunity for students to learn about the relationship between poverty, education, and health status (Campbell, Thompkins, & Westfall, 2002).

The initial intent was to offer this class, along with a booster course the following semester, to a large pool of 10th grade students interested in health careers. However, a timing problem necessitated alterations to the original plan. The Public Health Pipeline project leaders quickly regrouped. They restructured the course as a single elective offered to 11th and 12th graders and eliminated the booster course. The project partners contracted with a new instructor to teach the course (Campbell, Thompkins, & Westfall, 2002).

In its first year, the course attracted only seven students. The class met daily for a 90-minute block of time throughout the semester. Although there was no classroom available for the students, the small class size enabled them to meet in the library and computer lab. The flexibility of location provided opportunities for the students to conduct Internet and library research (Campbell, Thompkins, & Westfall, 2002).

The course design introduced students to five areas of public health: health service administration, biostatistics, epidemiology, behavioral sciences/health education, and environmental health services. Instruction included a combination of class lecture, computer research, guest speakers, and field trips. Eight guest speakers in the health field spoke to the students about their areas of expertise. The students learned about the impact of public health policies and government regulations on the restaurant business through tours of the school cafeteria and a local restaurant. One expert from the county sanitation office offered a food handler class. The class took field trips to water treatment plants to learn about water purification and sewage treatment. During a visit to the local university, students spoke with professors in health-related departments. Web-based research activities allowed students to gain deeper knowledge about the topics introduced by the guest speakers and field trips (Campbell, Thompkins, & Westfall, 2002).

Challenges
During the first two years, this project faced enormous upheaval because of staff turnover. The resignation of one of the project codirectors, who had been instrumental in the overall management and public relations for the project, posed a serious challenge. Although a replacement quickly stepped in, a void developed in the project's supervision and communication. Turnover in school superintendents compounded the situation, requiring renewed

effort to build support for the project with the new school district leader. One project champion, who had links to both the school and a local health care organization, helped keep the project afloat through these changes (Campbell, Thompkins, & Westfall, 2002).

The continuity of the project demonstrates that those involved remained flexible as they dealt with each challenge; however, these transitions took a toll on the overall success of the project. With attention focused on project management, staff did not effectively use feedback to strengthen the curriculum. They revised the list of guest speakers and field trips, expanded Web-based learning, and added a research paper requirement. Unfortunately, the changes did not provide students with a more in-depth experience of public health, nor did they offer opportunities for authentic student engagement.

Outcome

In the second year, an intern from West Virginia University assessed the effectiveness of the project. Students in the class took pre- and post-tests to measure how much they had learned about public health and their knowledge of careers in the field. Results at the end of the year showed insignificant gains in both areas. Students reported they did not feel adequately challenged and the course continued to lack depth (Campbell, Thompkins, & Westfall, 2002).

This project, in a community that could have benefited from a successful public health program, is an example of the need for assessment and the use of feedback early on and throughout a project to address concerns. When the project received substantial feedback at the end of the first year, the staff made some changes. However, these alterations proved to be inadequate. Staffing challenges affected the project's ability to be flexible throughout the course and to respond to ongoing assessment and feedback effectively. Information from a variety of sources could have been used to deepen the students' experiences, make the course more challenging, and strengthen connections with the community. Although the Public Health Pipeline project did not provide students with in-depth or rigorous learning experiences, it did meet one of its goals. Some students who completed the course decided to explore careers in health as a result of their participation the project (Campbell, Thompkins, & Westfall, 2002).

What We Learned:
Assessment and Review

1. What works best

◆ Ongoing assessment rather than a one time, year-end review helps address challenges as they surface. This will strengthen the project and does not necessarily take more time or energy if ongoing assessment is a part of the original plan and all the partners anticipate it.

◆ Use a variety of self-evaluation methods. Feedback from students is essential, either in daily reflection writings or regular feedback forms. Also gather feedback from other teachers, administrators, interns, and public health professionals. Videotaping the class is another form of feedback.

◆ Use the feedback you receive to make changes—feedback isn't useful if it's not used.

2. Flexibility

◆ Be flexible with planning and scheduling; realize things could change at the last minute.

◆ Have a Plan B and be willing to move on to it if necessary. Create Plan C if Plans A and B don't work.

◆ Train others who can easily step in if necessary. Backup staffing can be a real asset in a pinch.

◆ Keep the students' needs at the forefront. Remember you are doing this to provide them with a challenging, high-quality educational experience.

3. Common challenges

◆ There is never enough classroom time. The best way to deal with this is to set priorities, stay organized, and keep on top of scheduling changes caused by testing, assemblies, and field trips. Be realistic about what you can accomplish with the time you have.

◆ Keep schedule and class interruptions limited by communicating frequently with school administrators and project staff.

◆ Turnover is a common problem. Have backup teachers ready and trained. Establish a leadership succession in case project leaders leave unexpectedly. Be sure there are multiple champions to continue the project through staffing transitions.

◆ Don't focus exclusively on the problems. Be sure evaluations and feedback highlight successes.

8

Administrative Support

Key to Success: Administrative Support

The Health in Education Initiative found that strong administrative support facilitated success, continuity, and growth of the public health projects. Administrative support can provide access to resources. It can also reduce the time and effort that goes toward dealing with obstacles like schedule conflicts and class interruptions. A sense of team spirit develops when the administration is on board and energy is directed toward making the project work. With a new project there are many unknowns, and strong administrative support greatly eases the way.

Benefits of administrative support
◆ Access to resources
◆ Minimization of potential schedule conflicts and class interruptions
◆ Sense of team spirit
◆ Continuity of the project over time

Administrators control what happens at the school level, and without their support the continuity of any project is uncertain. After the ASCD Health in Education Initiative funding ended, the public health projects were more likely to continue if the school principal saw the value in the project. The principal either made the case for the project at the district level or had control of the budget and allocated school resources to keep the project going.

Even with strong initial support, however, tight budgets and staff turnover hinder some of the most successful endeavors. Anticipate the need to get support from new administrators at the school and in the district office. Several schools spent a lot of time and energy dealing with this challenge because they were not prepared for it. Keep good records of all assessments, evaluations, media clippings, and samples of student work. Ask partners or community members to send letters about the project to new administrators.

A public health project has a lot of assets, but it can be a tough sell in this era of standards and high-stakes testing. Develop a rigorous curriculum so that your project is not perceived as a disposable soft course. Linking it to health education requirements and other state standards makes a stronger academic case for your project. Gaining support from school and district administration will come more easily if the project fulfills mandatory requirements, supports the mission of the school, and boosts students' performance.

Taking the time to get support from the school principal and public health agency administrator is time well spent. Be clear and realistic about the type of support that you need. Ask for a specific commitment, explaining the benefits of your project to the school, the students, and the community. Understand that administrators may be concerned about the many priorities facing the school or agency. Gather your community or school health data and use the resources in this book to develop a rationale for your project. Plan your presentation to the administrators carefully and be prepared for difficult questions.

Once you have approval from the school and the public health agency, involve the administrators in appropriate ways. Have the principal kick off the project at a special event or assembly. Thank administrators for their support. Some Health in Education Initiative project staff found that mere verbal backing from administrators in the planning phase developed into significant support by communicating regularly about the project's successes and including the principal or public health administrator in key meetings or events.

Look to build other sources of support from within the school and the community. This can be particularly useful if political backing for the project is weak. Do not set the project apart from the school; make sure you see it as part of the school's mission and make that connection for others. If you've connected the project to state standards, share that information with school faculty. Garner support from your colleagues by inviting their feedback on the changes they may be seeing in students or about activities in which the students are participating. Help them see the connection between the project, student success, and community support for the school as a whole.

If the local health department or university is not involved, let them know what you are doing and specific ways they can assist and benefit from participation in the project. Talk about the project and attract attention to it. Write articles to the local paper, or better yet, let students from the project write articles to help spread the word about what they are doing for the community. Communicate every success along the way, even the small ones.

Sources of support for public health models
(1) Education
The district:
◆ Superintendent
◆ Deputy superintendent
◆ District health coordinator
◆ District curriculum coordinator

The school:
◆ Principal
◆ Vice principal
◆ School health coordinator
◆ School nurse
◆ School counselor
◆ Teachers
◆ Staff
◆ Students

◆ Parents with students at the school
◆ School health council members

(2) Public Health
◆ Administrators
◆ Health promotion/education staff
◆ Health care staff
◆ Public health board

(3) The Community
◆ Community organizations
◆ Universities with health or educator preparation programs
◆ Businesses
◆ Local media

Challenges

If administrative support seems unlikely or superficial, don't give up. Be flexible and find ways to integrate the project into something that already exists. Set priorities and revise the initial project plan and curriculum in a way that will still meet the goals. Build public relations for the project at every opportunity possible. There is a chance the administration will see the benefits or some unexpected source of support and resources will surface.

Ways to gain or maintain administrative support
◆ Create a rigorous curriculum that meets state and district standards.
◆ Integrate the project into the existing curriculum.
◆ Communicate every success.
◆ Spread the word in the community.
◆ Set priorities.
◆ Be flexible.
◆ Be persistent.

Community Health Leadership

McLean County High School, Green River District Health Department, and the McLean County Youth Services Center, Kentucky

Judy Martin is a veteran teacher at McLean County High School in Kentucky, with retirement right around the corner. Several years ago she got involved in teaching a new public health class for the school. She's excited by the course because of its interesting curriculum, field trips, guest speakers, and community service projects. It is a lot of extra work, but it all gets done with help from partners in the community.

The McLean County School District collaborated with the Green River Health Department and the McLean County Youth Services Center to create a course on public health for high school students. This partnership got the project off the ground, and nearly four years later the course continues to thrive as a result of this collaboration.

"I wouldn't be able to do this class without these partners," says Martin. A staff member with a strong background in health from the McLean County Youth Services Center developed the Community Health Leadership curriculum. At the beginning of each school year, the partners meet to go over the class schedule. The health department arranges field trips and guest speakers for the class, the Youth Services Center handles all the details and paperwork for any class activities outside the school, and Martin teaches the class. "It's a real partnership," she says. "I couldn't do all this on my own."

The model
The class targets high-performing students. The top 10 percent of the sophomore and junior classes receive a letter inviting them to participate in the class. In addition to class lectures, guest speakers, and field trips, throughout the semester students are given portfolio-writing assignments on public health topics and opportunities for self-assessment. Students also work in small groups to develop public health intervention presentations targeted at

younger children on one of five topics—alcohol and drugs, tobacco, sexuality, environment, and nutrition (Martin & Tucker, 2002).

The leadership component requires that each student perform 10 hours of community service work outside of class. While students initially complained about the community service hours, in the end many of them found that it helped them get college scholarships. The first year, the students gave a combined total of 225 hours in service to their community (Martin & Tucker, 2002).

Highlights of this model
◆ Class lecture
◆ Guest speakers
◆ Field trips
◆ Portfolio writing
◆ Opportunities for self-assessment
◆ Outreach presentations
◆ Community service

Challenges
Class interruptions, staffing changes, and lack of time to cover all the material are regular challenges facing the Community Health Leadership project. School budget constraints, however, have been the greatest obstacle. Financial issues threatened this project from the very beginning, even though there was initial district support. During the first year the district asked for justification of the project and at one point sought to divert funds for the course to pay for a school nurse. The project champions pointed out the intent of the project, the grant restrictions, and that the course helped students meet health education standards and fulfill the state writing standards. Students from the class performed well on skills tests for family and consumer science. In addition, the Community Health Leadership project gave students the opportunity to complete required community service work. These arguments made a strong case for the course. Once the district staff became more aware of the benefits of the class, the district stopped challenging its continuation (Martin & Tucker, 2002).

Outcome

In the first two years, the students in the Community Health Leadership class created age-appropriate intervention projects that educated more than 500 young children. Nearly 150 6th and 7th graders attended a 90-minute presentation entitled "Alcohol, Can You Handle It?" developed by one team of high school students. Another team targeted 3rd grade students for a presentation focused on good nutrition, "You Are What You Eat." Students also created a presentation called "Hand Washing Is Cool" for preschoolers. To keep the community informed, the Community Health Leadership students wrote articles for the local newspaper about their projects (Martin & Tucker, 2002).

Because these high school students served as role models for the younger students, it was important that the teenagers "walk the talk." In other words, if they chose to work on an alcohol presentation, they must not be drinkers. If they chose to work on a tobacco presentation, they must not be tobacco users themselves. One student from a farming family selected tobacco as his topic, even though growing tobacco was his family's livelihood. Through the class, the student developed an understanding about the dangers of tobacco and quit chewing it (Martin & Tucker, 2002).

Recognition of the students' intervention projects extended beyond the school and community. Students were invited to present their projects at the CDC-DASH National Leadership Conference and at the ASCD Annual Conference. Students also made a presentation to the national Family, Career and Community Leaders of America (FCCLA). Of 25 students enrolled in the class, 16 received recognition for their accomplishments by FCCLA (Martin & Tucker, 2002).

Assessments indicated that students' knowledge of public health increased and their personal communication and leadership skills improved. According to one evaluation, a quarter of the class expressed a desire to pursue health careers and one student attended a summer camp on health careers (Martin & Tucker, 2002).

Continuity and growth

As the Community Health Leadership project continued, it also evolved. This past year the students created a new intervention project—a one-day summit. After conducting research they decided to target 6th graders, because this is the age that children start to make decisions about drugs, alcohol, tobacco, sexuality, and nutrition. The Community Health Leadership students organized the entire event. They contacted the middle school principal, who agreed to hold the summit for all 166 students in the 6th grade. The high school Drug Club kicked off the event with a skit on drugs. Then, in rotating teams, the Community Health Leadership students taught different sessions on each of the five topics. The day culminated with a keynote speaker followed by a reflection time with healthy, low-fat snacks (Martin & Tucker, 2002).

This kind of hands-on education is what excites not only the high school students but also their teacher. "I love to see the kids doing things [in the school and community]," says instructor Martin. "It makes a big difference." She attributes the success of the project and its full enrollment to the way it engages the students. "The kids talk it up because of all the extra [activities] we do."

The administration can now clearly see the value in a challenging course that (1) elicits student engagement, (2) has a strong community outreach component, (3) fulfills a number of academic requirements, and (4) gained national recognition. The school principal is very pleased and has given the course instructor carte blanche. With such strong support, Martin has deferred her retirement for several more years so that she can continue teaching this important class (Martin & Tucker, 2002).

Future Shock: Practicum in Public Health Research

Cambridge Public Schools, Health of the City, and the Cambridge Department of Public Health, Massachusetts

NOTE: More information on this project is in Chapter 6: Student Engagement in the Community.

Four teachers from the Cambridge Rindge and Latin School in Massachusetts collaborated with Harvard University's public health faculty to conceptualize and develop a public health curriculum for high school students. This took place at a professional development workshop held during the summer. The four high school teachers—from mathematics, humanities, history, and science—formed an interdisciplinary teaching team for the semester-long course. Despite the cost of putting four teachers in one classroom, the deputy superintendent supported the project (Grady, 2002).

The Future Shock curriculum contained a strong research focus that required students to understand statistics. Because of the math component many students considered the course difficult; however, this rigorous element attracted a number of good students. The first time it was offered, the course quickly filled up with 30 juniors and seniors. The students rose to the challenge of developing their own public health research projects. Interdisciplinary collaboration worked well among the four teachers, who also shared responsibility for managing the sizable quantity of work the student projects entailed (Grady, 2002).

With such success, the teachers intended to offer Future Shock again the following year. Budget issues and staff turnover, however, made them change their plan. When the deputy superintendent left the school system, the project lost its primary administrative backer. Without champions in the district, the future of the class teetered (Grady, 2002).

"We lost political support, and so we were thrown into a 'make-do' mode to keep the course alive," writes Elizabeth Grady (2002), the school-based project director. This illustrates that a successful program can be vulnerable when it lacks administrative support at the district level. It became necessary to rethink the course in order to keep the project going.

Adaptability

The principal, the course instructors, and the students wanted to see Future Shock continue. However, budget cuts allowed for only one instructor. This presented a challenge, because the original design required a team of teachers to adequately assist the students with the implementation of their projects and to provide interdisciplinary collaboration. With the cut in staff, the instructor's workload would increase, there would be no collaboration across subject areas, and students would get less individual attention with their projects (Grady, 2002).

Meanwhile, the school began to look outside the district for additional support and resources. They applied for, and received, the ASCD Health in Education Initiative grant to pay for a Future Shock instructor. A former teacher from the initial interdisciplinary team, familiar with the course content, agreed to step in and teach the course for a year. As required by the grant application, the project staff developed a partnership with the local public health department, which played an important part in maintaining the continuity of the course. The health department supplied speakers on relevant topics, wrote up local public health cases for the students to study, and created mentoring and summer internships for students.

Staff also made revisions to the curriculum. With just one teacher, they had to change the way the course material would be covered to allow ample time for the student projects. Changes to the course schedule meant that once the students had a good understanding of public health, class instruction decreased from five to three days per week so students could begin to work on their research projects (Grady, 2002).

Although the course design changed, Future Shock continued to be rigorous. Students developed authentic research projects that culminated in a public presentation to parents, other classes, school and district officials, and the local health organization. Through word of mouth the course became so popular that by the fourth year, at the students' request, it was offered both semesters (Grady, 2002).

A new model
The project staff hoped to see Future Shock continue once ASCD Health in Education Initiative funding ended. However, reliance on district funding and existing teachers remains a challenge. This past year, Future Shock could not be offered because there was no instructor available (Grady, 2002).

The local health department may offer a viable solution for the reinstitution of the project. Aware of the school's budget constraints and impressed by the quality of the students' work, a staff member from Cambridge Alliance of Health has offered to teach the course. This might be the next step in the evolution of this project. Success, however, will depend on support from the school. An ideal scenario would be a team-teaching arrangement with school and public health staff working together during a transition period.

With the trend in budget cuts for education and social services, schools and public health departments may need to rely more heavily on one another. "In these tightened financial times we're seeing more collaborations developing in this city," says Grady. Looking down the road, she envisions the course becoming a feeder for senior internships. It will expose students to an authentic educational experience in public health while simultaneously providing the health department with a pool of potential employees.

Obstacles
◆ Loss of administrative support at the district level
◆ Budget cuts requiring alterations to the original course design
◆ Lack of available instructors

Coping strategies
◆ Remain adaptable.
◆ Persevere.
◆ Think creatively.
◆ Revise the way the curriculum is presented.
◆ Look for other sources of support and additional resources.
◆ Rely more heavily on community organizations and agencies.

What We Learned:
Administrative Support

1. Things you can do to build support
◆ Use the program to meet state standards or career training requirements. With heightened attention on state standards and accountability nationwide, this helps make the case for the project and gain support from the school and district administrators.

◆ Make the curriculum rigorous. Develop research-based concepts.

◆ Involve district, school, and public health administrators in appropriate ways: special events, assemblies, and meetings.

◆ Ask school staff for feedback about changes they may be seeing in students or about activities in which the students are participating in order to elicit school support.

◆ Communicate with local businesses, agencies, and universities not involved in the project to build their interest in it.

◆ Inform parents about the project and its successes to gain their support.

◆ Use publicity to attract attention to the project—draw in the local media. Have the students write articles for the local newspaper.

◆ Share every success along the way, even the small ones.

2. **Common challenges**

◆ When administrative support seems unlikely or superficial, don't give up. Gather your community or school health data and use the resources in this book to develop a rationale for your project.

◆ You will need to get support from new administrators at the school and in the district office. Be prepared for this and don't let it catch you off guard. Keep good records of your project assessments and evaluations to show them, along with any media clippings of the project and photos or projects your students have completed. Ask your partners or involved parents to send new administrators letters on behalf of the project.

◆ Unsupportive colleagues at school can be a problem, especially if administrative support is weak. Help school staff see the connection between the project and student success and community support for the school as a whole.

9

Getting Started

Keys to Success: Commitment, Professional Development, and Resources

Commitment

A public health project requires a personal commitment. Your passion will be the engine that drives you to do the work to get started. As the models in this book demonstrate, a project cannot be done effectively by just one person. Use your belief in the project to rally the enthusiasm and energy of others in your school, district, and community.

Support your passion for the project with data indicating why it is necessary. Make your case by demonstrating the link between health and education and the relationship between poor health and poor academic outcomes. Examine available data on the health of students in your school or community. Use these data to show the specific health challenges your students face and identify gaps in the school or district's current health plan. Explain the benefits of a public health curriculum and how it will fill a gap or enhance existing health or educational programs.

People are often more receptive when a project seems feasible. Once the gaps and the needs of the school are identified, brainstorm ways to make the project work. Think about how it can be done without adding staff or classroom space. Consider what other community agencies and institutions can contribute to the project.

It might take longer than you anticipate to gain support from school or district staff. Even if you are passionate about the project, the data show there's a need, and it seems doable, others may still have apprehensions. Give them time to absorb the ideas you've presented. Be sure you understand their concerns and explore ways to overcome them. Wait several weeks to approach the subject again. Be patient and don't give up.

Professional Development

Teachers may have strong instructional skills but need training in public health and service learning. Public health professionals have experience and knowledge of health issues but often need training in instruction and classroom management. It is important to acknowledge staff strengths and limitations early on.

As with most new projects, problems will arise if adequate professional development does not occur. The Health in Education Initiative found that when teachers designed and taught the curriculum without adequate training in public health, they had trouble integrating the material into the class and difficulty developing effective service learning experiences for the students. On the other hand, when public health professionals or university staff taught the class or curriculum, they often encountered challenges dealing with classroom management issues and student accountability. Base your professional development plan on the experience of the people involved.

Common topics to be addressed in professional development
◆ Classroom management
◆ Student accountability
◆ Curriculum development and integration
◆ Public health versus medicine
◆ Public health issues in the community
◆ Effective service learning activities

Ways to support professional development
◆ Find experts to target professional development.
◆ Link up with other schools.

- Share resources.
- Provide extra classroom support.
- Teach in teams.

Professional development for school personnel might focus on (1) developing an appropriate curriculum, (2) learning the fundamentals of public health, (3) understanding the specific public health issue(s) in the community, and (4) developing effective service learning activities. Targeted professional development can come from project partners or experts within the community. Schools might also be able to tap into district-level support or link up with other schools that are doing similar projects to share resources and training.

If university or public health professionals plan to teach the curriculum, the school should be prepared to provide extra classroom support. The teachers know their students' strengths and weaknesses, so be sure to talk about potential challenges and how to effectively deal with them. Consider a team-teaching situation, especially at the beginning, to address class management and student accountability problems that arise.

Resources
With school districts and public health agencies facing budget cuts, obtaining outside funding might increase the feasibility of getting a new project started. All of the school models described in this book received a $20,000 grant each year for two years. In some cases, the grant budget covered materials and field trips. In other cases, it paid for instructors and project coordinators. Several schools were able to pool resources from a variety of sources, allowing their projects to continue beyond the Health in Education Initiative funding period.

External funding came with stipulations that proved to be beneficial in a number of ways. Accountability requirements helped keep the projects on track. Although specific criteria had to be met, there was also a certain degree of flexibility in how each project could be carried out. An experiential component added depth to the curriculum, providing students with opportunities for engagement in the community, an authentic experience of public health, and exposure to careers in the field. The requirement to form partnerships resulted in collaborations among schools/districts, public health agencies, and universities that had not previously existed in some communities. Given the fiscal crises facing education and public health, these relationships will be increasingly important for meeting community needs in the years to come.

Pros and cons of funding sources:

◆ External funding

Pros: Helps get a project off the ground; institutes accountability.

Cons: May jeopardize continuity of a project when funding ends

◆ Existing funds

Pros: Facilitates longevity of a project; energy can be put into project development rather than fund raising.

Cons: Are potentially limited and may dry up with budget cuts.

When considering additional funding, first determine whether the district already receives money to fund new projects. If there is money, find out if it is distributed directly to the school for discretionary use. This might be a good source to tap before looking for external support. If, however, the district has no existing money for this purpose, determine if your school district is eligible to receive funding for new projects in health, service learning, or community projects and if the school is allowed to pursue such funding on its own (Fetro, 1998).

Specific project goals helped some of the Health in Education Initiative projects access other sources of funding. Several projects leveraged their grant money to receive additional state and local funding through the health department, school district, or community funds. For example, a project that focused on physical activity and nutrition tapped into the state health department's cardiovascular health funding. Other projects found financial support or staff through school-to-career funding, service learning funds, Safe and Drug Free Schools budgets, youth development programs, and adolescent pregnancy prevention programs.

Projects found that they could also receive in-kind services and other resources from community agencies and businesses. Such resources can free up funds or staff time and should not be overlooked. Local businesses donated food for special events held by many of the projects, and one school received refurbished exercise equipment for a faculty wellness program. Although seeking donations took staff time, the results were worth the effort. Donors became champions for the project and learned more about the school and its efforts. In some cases, once the project became well-known in the community, businesses and organizations approached the project directors with offers of assistance and resources. Be sure to recognize your donors in some way—a thank you note from the students, a certificate, or a mention in a newspaper article may be appropriate. It is also important to understand your school and district policies about donations. Keep issues of commercialism and conflict-of-interest in mind when seeking or accepting donations.

Projects that use existing resources in the school, district, and community and do not depend exclusively on outside funding may be better off in the long run. Too great a reliance on external funding, particularly for the larger expenses of instruction and project management, can jeopardize the longevity of a project. ASCD found that if the school, district, or another community organization did not ultimately absorb costs when the Health in Education Initiative grant funding ended, the project was not likely to continue.

It is critical to approach your project with goals based on financial realities. This, along with a clear understanding of the professional development needs, will start the project off on the right foot. Enthusiasm for and commitment to the project at all stages will also contribute greatly to its success.

10

Final Comments

A public health curriculum dependent on community partnerships is a relatively novel concept. Most of the schools cited in this book ventured into unknown territory to develop a new curriculum model, and in doing so discovered an enriching and rewarding experience for both students and teachers. Students were generally enthusiastic about the subject and eager to help address the public health problems in their schools and communities, and teachers were excited to try something new.

A public health partnership project is good for schools and students in a number of different ways. Students learn information about health that they can use and skills that they can transfer to other topics. As several Health in Education Initiative projects discovered, the partnership can also motivate students to consider higher education. Student engagement in the school and community fosters student connectedness, which can improve students' academic outcomes and behaviors. When students develop an understanding of their role in the community, schools meet their civic mission, and community support for the school can improve. Some projects also experienced increased teacher satisfaction and retention.

The schools that participated in the Health in Education Initiative represent a broad spectrum of educational environments across the country: urban and rural, racially diverse and homogenous, large and small, high poverty and more economically balanced. The contexts in which each curriculum model developed also varied greatly. Some schools fit the model into an existing School-to-Work program, and others developed a new curriculum. Some sought out the top students, and others included all levels. Class sizes varied from 7 to more than 50 students. All the schools addressed different public health issues.

Through these projects, the Health in Education Initiative learned there are many variables that can affect success. A positive outcome depends in large part on the strength of the partnerships, multiple champions, infrastructure support, focus on a single topic, strong student engagement in the community, ongoing assessment and review, and administrative support.

Because of the differences at each project site, success was measured in different ways. The benefits were both tangible and intangible. In Rhode Island, the Lead Smarts project helped address a serious community health issue; and attesting to its success, the project received an award for Excellence in Public Health Promotion from the Rhode Island Department of Health. In Washington, the project exposed new immigrants to careers in public health, where ethnic diversity is desperately needed. In Utah, the PATHS project's public health approach improved attitudes toward personal health among students and faculty and also had a positive impact on students' self-esteem.

A public health curriculum with a service learning component teaches students how to apply what they learn in a concrete way that makes a contribution to their school and community. Education's mission is to provide youth with a foundation they can use to serve society. The ASCD Health in Education Initiative demonstrated that students, schools, and communities all reap rewards from a partnership between education and public health that prepares students to become responsible citizens.

References

Allen, L., Hogan, C., & Steinberg, A. (1998). *Knowing and doing: Connecting learning and work*. Providence, RI: Brown University.

Allen, R. (2002, March). Preparing for a healthy tomorrow. *Education Update, 44*(2), 4.

Allen, R. (2003). The democratic aims of service learning. *Educational Leadership, 60*(6), 51–54.

Association of Schools of Public Health. (2003). What is public health: What is public health practice. Retrieved March 17, 2003, from http://www.asph.org

Association of Schools of Public Health [Electronic bulletin board]. (2001). The population approach to public health. Reprinted with permission. Retrieved June 13, 2003, from http://www.asph.org/document .cfm?page=724

Bandura, A., Barbaranelli, C., Caprara, G. V., & Pastorelli, C. (2001). Self-efficacy beliefs as shapers of children's aspirations and career trajectories. *Child Development, 72*(1), 187–206.

Battistich, V., & Hom, A. (1997, December). The relationship between students' sense of their school as a community and their involvement in problem behaviors. *American Journal of Public Health, 87*(12), 1997–2001.

Billig, S. H. (2000). Research on K-12 school-based service learning: The evidence builds. *Phi Delta Kappan 81*(9), 658–664.

Blum, R. W., Beuhring, T., & Rinehart, P. M. (2000). *Protecting teens: Beyond race, income, and family structure*. (Available from Center For Adolescent Health, University of Minnesota, 200 Oak Street S.E., Suite 260, Minneapolis, MN 55455-2007)

Blum, R. W., & Rinehart, P. M. (1998). *Reducing the risk: Connections that make a difference in the lives of youth* [Monograph]. Minneapolis, MN: Division of General Pediatrics and Adolescent Health, Department of Pediatrics, University of Minnesota.

Campbell, L., Thompkins, N., & Westfall, L. J. (2002). *Mountaineer public health pipeline.* Unpublished report.

Carnegie Council on Adolescent Development. (1989). *Turning points: Preparing American youth for the 21st century.* A report of the Task Force on Education of Youth Adolescents. New York: Carnegie Corporation.

Carter, G. R. (2003, April 2). Is it good for the kids? Helping kids create healthier communities. *Education Week,* p. 28. [advertorial]

Centers for Disease Control and Prevention, School Health Policies and Programs Study (SHPPS). (2001). Percentage of states and districts requiring schools to teach health education by school level. Retrieved April 7, 2003, from http://www.cdc.gov/nccdphp/dash/shpps/factsheets/fs01_health_education.htm

Checkley, K. (2000, Spring). Health education. *Curriculum Update.*

Curtis, D. (2002, September). The power of projects. *Educational Leadership* 60(1), 50–53.

Deutsch, C. (2000, March). Common cause: School health & school reform. *Educational Leadership,* 57(6), 8–12.

Drake, M. V., & Lowenstein, D. H. (1998). The role of diversity in the health care needs of California. *Western Journals of Medicine, 168*(5), 348–354.

Dryfoos, J. G. (1994). *Full service schools: A revolution in health and social services for children, youth, and families.* San Francisco: Jossey-Bass.

Elhard, D. & Lavalier, K. (2002). *Community health awareness through teens.* Unpublished report.

Fetro, J. V. (1998). Implementing coordinated school health programs in local schools. In E. Marx, S. F. Wooley, & D. Northrup (Eds.). *Health is academic* (pp. 15–42). New York: Teachers College Press.

Fineberg, H. (1990). Public health vs. medicine. *The population approach to public health.* Harvard University School of Public Health. Reprinted with permission. Retrieved on March 13, 2003 from http://www.asph.org/document.cfm?page=724

Fleming, R. (2002). *Cross-cultural education in public health.* Unpublished report.

Gast, J., & Lounsbery, M. (2002). *The planned adolescent approach to community health: An integrated school curriculum.* Unpublished report.

Glickman, C. D. (2003). *Holding sacred ground: Essays on leadership, courage, and endurance in our schools.* San Francisco: Jossey-Bass.

Grady, E. (2002). *Future shock: Practicum in public health research skills for health activism.* Unpublished report.

Grunbaum, J. A., Kann, L., Kinchen, S. A., Williams, B., Ross, J. G., Lowry, R., et al. (2002, June 28). Youth risk behavior surveillance: United States 2001. *Morbidity and Mortality Weekly Report, 51*(SS04), 1–64. Retrieved June 19, 2003, from http://www.cdc.gov/mmwr/preview/mmwrhtml/ss5104a1.htm

Hawkins, D. J., & Catalano, R. F. (1990). Broadening the vision of education: Schools as health promoting environments. *Journal of School Health, 60*(4), 178–181.

Joint Committee on National Health Education Standards. (1995). *National health education standards: Achieving health literacy.* Atlanta, GA: American Cancer Society. Reprinted with permission.

Kinsey, K. K., & Walker, A. (2002). *Healthy me + healthy you = healthy schools and healthy neighborhoods.* Unpublished report.

Kolbe, L. J. (1990). An epidemiological surveillance system to monitor the prevalence of youth behaviors that most affect health. *Health Education, 21*(3), 44–48.

Kolbe, L. J., Kann, L., & Brener, N. D. (2001). Overview and summary of findings: School health policies and programs study 2000. *Journal of School Health, 71*(7), 253–259.

Kozol, J. (1991). *Savage inequalities: Children in America's schools.* New York: Crown Publishers.

Larabee, J. W. (Ed.). (1749/1961). *The papers of Benjamin Franklin* (Vol. 3, p. 442). New Haven, CT: Yale University Press.

Learning First Alliance. (2001, November). *Every child learning: Safe and supportive schools.* (Available from Association for Supervision and Curriculum Development, P.O. Box 79760, Baltimore, MD 21279-0760)

Martin, J. & Tucker, J. (2002). *Community health leadership.* Unpublished report.

Marx, E., Wooley, S. F., & Northrop, D. (Eds.). (1998). *Health is academic: A guide to coordinated school health programs.* New York: Teachers College Press.

National Commission on Service-Learning. (2002). *Learning in deed: The power of service learning for American schools.* Battle Creek, MI: W. K. Kellogg Foundation. Reprinted with permission. Retrieved May 16, 2003, from http://www.servicelearning.org/article/archive/35

National Service Learning Cooperative. (1998). *Essential elements of service-learning.* (Available from National Youth Leadership Council, 1667 Snelling Avenue North, St. Paul, MN 55108)

Novello, A. C., Degraw, C., & Kleinman, D. V. (1992, January). Healthy children ready to learn: An essential collaboration between health and education. *U.S. Department of Health and Human Services, Public Health Reports, 107*(1), 3–15.

O'Byrne, D. World Health Organization. Retrieved January 11, 2001, from http://www.who.int/en

Public Health Functions Steering Committee. Public Health in America (Fall, 1994). Retrieved March 17, 2002, from http://www.health .gov/phfunctions

Resnick, M. D., Bearman, P. S., Blum, R. W., Bauman, K. E., Harris, K. M., Jones, J., et al. (1997). Protecting adolescents from harm: Findings from the national longitudinal study on adolescent health. *Journal of the American Medical Association, 178*(10), 823–832.

Rhode Island Department of Health. (2002). *Lead poisoning in Rhode Island: The numbers.* Providence, RI: Author.

Rhode Island Kids Count. (2002). *2002 Rhode Island kids count fact book.* Retrieved April 14, 2003, from http://www.rikidscount.org/rikc/ LinksPage.asp?PageID=201&PageName=2002Factbook

Rhode Island Kids Count. (2003). *2003 Rhode Island kids count fact book.* Retrieved April 14, 2003, from http://www.rikidscount.org/rikc/ MultiPiecePage.asp?PageID=267&PageName=2003FBInd

Roberts, L., Cordero, C., & Pichardo, C. (2002). *College exploratory program in public health.* Unpublished report.

Rose, L. C., & Gallup, A. M. (2000, September). The 32nd annual Phi Delta Kappa/Gallup Poll of the public's attitudes toward the public schools. *Phi Delta Kappan, 82*(1), 41–57. Available: http://www.pdkintl .org/kappan/kpol0009.htm

Saldivar, C. & Tapper, S. (2002). *Students teaching other peers.* Unpublished report.

Toole, J. & Toole, P. (1995). Reflection as a tool for turning service experiences into learning experiences. In C. W. Kinsley & K. McPherson (Eds.). *Enriching the curriculum through service learning* (pp. 99–114). Alexandria, VA: Association for Supervision and Curriculum Development.

U.S. Census Bureau. (2000a). Population Projections Program. *Projections of the total resident population by 5-year age groups, race, and Hispanic origin with special age categories: Middle series, 2006 to 2010.* Retrieved May 2, 2003, from http://landview.census.gov/population/projections/nation/ summary/np-t4-c.txt

U.S. Census Bureau. (2000b). Population Division. *The foreign-born population in the United States.* Retrieved June 13, 2003, from http://www.census.gov/ prod/2000pubs/p20-534.pdf

U.S. Census Bureau. (2001). Population Division. *Measurement of net international migration to the United States: 1990 to 2000.* Retrieved March 17, 2002, from http://www.census.gov/population/www/documentation/ twps0051.html

U.S. Department of Education. (2001). National Center for Education Statistics. Table 6 – Percent of the population 3 to 34 years old enrolled in school, by age: April 1940 to October 2000. Retrieved April 7, 2003, from http://nces.ed.gov/pubs2002/digest2001/tables/ dt006.asp

U.S. Department of Health and Human Services. (1999). *Mental health: A report of the Surgeon General.* Rockville, MD: U.S. Department of Health and Human Services, Substance Abuse and Mental Health Services Administration, Center for Mental Health Services, National Institutes of Health, National Institute of Mental Health. Retrieved April 24, 2003, from http://www.surgeongeneral.gov/library/ mentalhealth/chapter3/sec1.html

U.S. Department of Health and Human Services. (2000, November). *Healthy people 2010: Understanding and improving health* (2nd ed.). Washington, DC: U.S. Government Printing Office. Retrieved March 20, 2003, from http://www.healthypeople.gov/Document/ tableofcontents.htm

Weitzman, M., & DuPleiss, H. M. (1997). Health care for children of immigrant families. *Pediatrics, 100*(1), 153–157.

Witmer, J. T., & Anderson, C. S. (1994). *How to establish a high school service learning program.* Alexandria, VA: Association for Supervision and Curriculum Development.

Wooler, R. & Herman, A. (2002). *Lead smarts. Unpublished report.*

Appendix

These 10 sites received grant funding from March 2000 through June 2002 to develop and sustain school-community public health partnerships.

Cambridge Public Schools with Health of the City and the Cambridge Department of Public Health, Massachusetts

Future Shock: Practicum in Public Health Research Skills for Health Activism

Future Shock provided students with in-depth, project-based learning. Students learned and practiced public health skills through mathematics, social studies, language arts, and science. They applied the methodologies of social and behavioral science through projects, service learning opportunities, and student internships. The Future Shock curriculum included an exploration of the ethical and legal issues encountered in public health. The students presented their results to the school, public health agency staff, and the community.

Grand Rapids High School with the Itasca County Resource Center, Minnesota

Community Health Awareness Through Teens (CHAT)

The CHAT program operated in the school's public health and community issues course. Public health staff served as mentors for the students as they researched five community public health issues. Through community service and service learning activities, the students participated in delivering health promotion information and programs related to each of the five public health issues. Students also developed education programs about environmental health. They learned about developing and broadcasting health messages through the media. They also created a video about the impact of public health issues on everyday life.

McLean County High School with McLean County Youth Services Center and the Green River District Health Department, Kentucky

A Community Health Leadership Proposal

The program developers created a public health primer as coursework for the community health youth leaders. The course in public health leadership taught the youth leaders basic concepts, problem solving, and critical thinking skills needed to make informed decisions. The community health youth leaders prepared and implemented public health education activities in schools and the community. They also participated in community service activities and field trips to public health-related facilities. The youth leaders made their work meaningful to the community by focusing their research on public health issues identified in the county public health statistics.

Pawtucket School District with the Rhode Island Youth Guidance Center, Memorial Hospital, and the Department of Health, Rhode Island

Lead Smarts

Through lead awareness classes, classroom projects, certification classes, and internships, high school students learned about lead and educated the community about lead as an environmental hazard that affects health and human development. A multidisciplinary project team developed a curriculum on lead that highlighted the community public health professions involved in the issue. A wide range of high school students participated in hands-on, community-connected learning: those in family and consumer science classes, ESL classes, school-to-career and special education classes, child development classes, and parenting classes for pregnant teens. The ESL students developed lead education brochures in the their languages of origin, as well as lead poisoning awareness posters and videotapes in various languages. During Year 2 of the project, teachers integrated lead education across the curriculum.

Belmont-Redwood Shores School District with the San Mateo County Public Health Education Program and the Department of Health Education at San Francisco State University, California

Students Teaching Other Peers (STOP)

STOP fostered awareness of public health issues and careers among middle and elementary school students and their teachers through a model peer education program. University health education majors provided training and support to middle school peer educators. The middle school students developed materials and curriculum for an asset-building and resiliency curriculum for 3rd graders. The middle school students presented health education lessons once a week for 10 weeks. They also participated in Public Health Week activities.

Ritchie County Schools with Ritchie County Primary Care Association and the Department of Community Medicine at West Virginia University, West Virginia

West Virginia Public Health Pipeline

The West Virginia Public Health Pipeline project introduced students to public health issues and careers through an interdisciplinary approach. A public health course enabled students to explore biostatistics, epidemiology, environmental health sciences, health sciences administration, and social and behavioral sciences. Learning strategies included interactive sessions with guest speakers, field trips, Web-based learning, student projects, and booster sessions. Students focused on public health issues facing their rural community and the impact of economics on public health. An advisory committee of public health practitioners and researchers guided the project.

Seattle School District with Seattle and King County Public Health, Washington

Cross-Cultural Education in Public Health

This project focused on providing immigrant students with a basic understanding of public health methods, language, and skills, encouraging student interest in public health careers. The public health course—presented to middle and high school ESL classes—included activities through which students could develop leadership skills. The cultural education component enabled students to examine health practices from a variety of viewpoints to facilitate the development of cultural sensitivity and competence. Students contributed to a health Web site focused on ethnic minority health issues. An end-of-the-year event brought together a variety of community organizations to examine ways that they could work together to further the efforts begun by this project.

Skyview High School and North Cache 8-9 Center School with Utah State University and Utah Department of Health, Utah

The Planned Approach to Healthier Schools (PATHS): An Integrated School Curriculum

Directors of PATHS developed an adaptation of the Centers for Disease Control and Prevention's model approach to community health promotion for use as a school-based curriculum for grades 9–12. Students at a middle school and a high school developed public health interventions to promote increased physical activity and healthy nutrition. Through the integration of public health-related assignments across the curriculum, students learned about health behavior change theory and designed a social marketing program called Get Up, Get Out, Get Fit. The curriculum included opportunities for students to develop creative problem-solving and decision-making skills and to learn the principles of communication, negotiation, data collection, and analysis. They also learned how to write for the media and conduct news conferences. The project included a teacher development component. Faculty developed a staff fitness program as a result of this project. At one school, the community has access to the fitness facility after school hours.

Thurgood Marshall Elementary School and La Salle Neighborhood Nursing Center, Pennsylvania

Healthy Me + Healthy You = Healthy Schools and Healthy Neighborhoods

This project included in-school, after-school, and summer camp components. During the first year of the project, public health topics and careers were integrated into the health curriculum, and related projects were carried out during after-school activities. The summer camp, held at La Salle University, focused on environmental health. In Year 2, the impact of the environment on health was included in the science classes. Middle-school students developed a public health book they used to teach kindergarten and 1st-grade students. The middle-school students learned about community resources and compiled them into a reference for teachers, students, and parents. Middle-school students also developed public service announcements for use on cable television.

William Howard Taft High School with Bronx-Lebanon Hospital and the Urban Public Health Program at Hunter College, New York

College Exploratory Program in Public Health

Students who enrolled in this project participated in a college campus–based course on Saturday mornings for 20 weeks, designed to increase their awareness of the public health field while improving their academic skills and preparedness for college. The students worked in teams to develop public health interventions. During the first year, these interventions focused on rodent control and sexually transmitted disease prevention. During Year 2, the students worked with the National Cancer Institute's Cancer Information Service to develop a tobacco-use prevention campaign targeted at Latino adolescents in New York City.

Sample Forms
and Tools

Sample forms and materials used by the projects in developing and sustaining their work.

- ◆ Partnerships chart—Lead Smarts
- ◆ Program design chart—Lead Smarts
- ◆ Example of local data—West Virginia Public Health Pipeline
- ◆ Selecting a focus and criteria for determining priority—Planned Approach to Healthier Schools (PATHS)
- ◆ Community action plan proposal—Community Health Awareness Through Teens (CHAT)
- ◆ Public health intervention work plan—Planned Approach to Healthier Schools (PATHS)
- ◆ Example of integrating a public health issue into various disciplines—Future Shock: Practicum in Public Health
- ◆ Service learning reflection activities—From *Enriching the Curriculum Through Service Learning*
- ◆ Rubric for evaluators—Community Health Awareness Through Teens (CHAT)
- ◆ Closing activity—College Exploratory Program in Public Health
- ◆ Outreach Outcomes—Lead Smarts

Lead Smarts Partnerships

During the 2002/2003 Academic Year

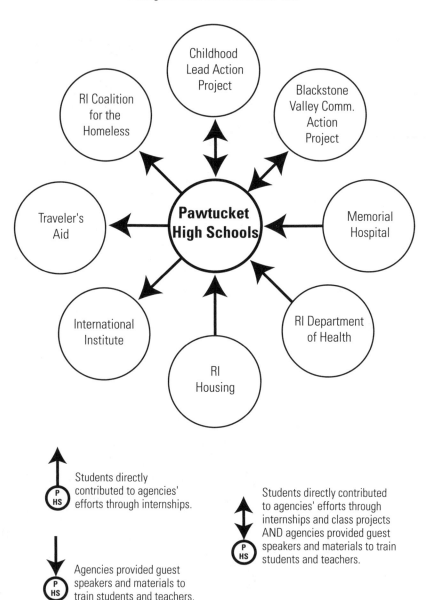

(Wooler & Herman, 2002)

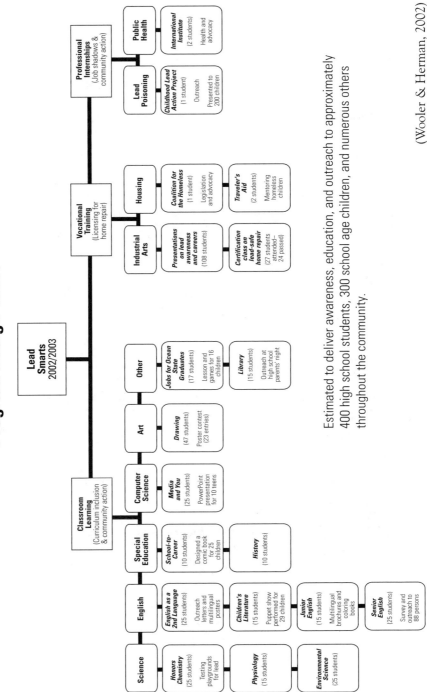

Program Design Chart

Lead Smarts 2002/2003

Classroom Learning (Curriculum inclusion & community action)

- **Science**
  - *Honors Chemistry* (25 students) — Testing playgrounds for lead
  - *Physiology* (15 students)
  - *Environmental Science* (25 students)
- **English**
  - *English as a 2nd Language* (25 students) — Outreach letters and multilingual posters
  - *Children's Literature* (15 students) — Puppet show performed for 29 children
  - *Junior English* (15 students) — Multilingual brochures and coloring books
  - *Senior English* (25 students) — Survey and outreach to 88 persons
- **Special Education**
  - *School-to-Career* (10 students) — Designed a comic book for 25 children
  - *History* (10 students)
- **Computer Science**
  - *Media and You* (25 students) — PowerPoint presentation for 10 teens
- **Art**
  - *Drawing* (47 students) — Poster contest (23 entries)
- **Other**
  - *Jobs for Ocean State Graduates* (17 students) — Lesson and games for 16 children
  - *Library* (15 students) — Outreach at high school parents' night

Vocational Training (Licensing for home repair)

- **Industrial Arts**
  - *Presentations on lead awareness and careers* (108 students)
  - *Certification class on lead-safe home repair* (27 students attended—24 passed)
- **Housing**
  - *Coalition for the Homeless* (1 student) — Legislation and advocacy
  - *Traveler's Aid* (2 students) — Mentoring homeless children

Professional Internships (Job shadows & community action)

- **Lead Poisoning**
  - *Childhood Lead Action Project* (1 student) — Outreach Presented to 200 children
- **Public Health**
  - *International Institute* (2 students) — Health and advocacy

Estimated to deliver awareness, education, and outreach to approximately 400 high school students, 300 school age children, and numerous others throughout the community.

(Wooler & Herman, 2002)

Example of Local Data

1997 Ritchie County Behavior Prevalences
Compared to 1992 Ritchie County and Estimated 1997 U.S. Prevalences

Category	1992 County Percent	1997 County Percent	SI*	1997 Estimated U.S. Percent	% Differences 1997 County from 1997 U.S.	SI*	County Rank
Physical Inactivity	46.9	51.1		29.7	72.0	*	7
Obesity	10.2	22.7	TS	17.0	33.7	*	14
Hypertension	25.7	22.0		23.3	−5.6		32
Seatbelt Nonuse	44.8	31.2	*	27.0	15.4		16
Cigarette Smoking	27.0	32.9		23.0	43.1	*	4
Smokeless Tobacco Use	8.0	13.2	TS	3.7	256.9	*	4
Binge Drinking	10.0	6.7	TS	13.5	TS	TS	28
No Health Insurance Ages 18–64	32.8	36.1		16.9	113.3	*	1
Difficulty Seeing Dr. Because of Cost	18.9	19.9		10.6	87.5	*	6

An asterisk (*) indicates a statistically significant difference from the U.S. rate.

SI: Significance indicator.

TS: Number is too small for a valid comparison.

Note: 1992 represents aggregated data from 1990–94.

     1997 represents aggregated data from 1995–99.

Note: The U.S. percent for physical inactivity is for 1996 due to lack of data for 1997.

Note: West Virginia's seatbelt use law went into effect on September 1, 1993.

Note: The range for county ranks in this column is 1 to 36.

Note: Two or more counties were grouped together to obtain an appropriate sample size.

Tables extracted from West Virginia County Health Profiles—2000.

(Campbell, Thompkins & Westfall, 2002)

Selecting a Focus

Criteria for Determining Priority

Importance
◆ Change will make a difference.
◆ Health problems have serious consequences for the community.

Changeability
◆ Behavior can be voluntarily changed.

Ways to Assess Importance

◆ Is the behavior widespread?
◆ Is the prevalence higher than that for the state or nation?
◆ Are the consequences serious?
◆ Are the behavior and the problem closely related?

Ways to Assess Changeability

◆ Behaviors are still in developmental stages.
◆ Behaviors are superficially tied to lifestyle.
◆ Behaviors are successfully changed in other programs.
◆ Literature suggests that the behaviors can be changed.

Setting Priorities

Use this matrix to determine which of the issues you are selecting are both important and changeable.

	Important	Less Important
Changeable		
Less Changeable		

(Gast & Lounsberry, 2002)

Community Action Plan Proposal

LARGE TOPIC AREA: _____

GROUP MEMBERS: _____

PART I: OUTLINE OF WORK

A. Identify the major problem/issue your action team will address.

B. Identify the target population(s) you will serve.

C. Describe a team vision for how things will look after your action plan is completed.

D. Identify what you expect to learn from this project.

E. Identify any factors that may be a potential obstacle in reaching your vision.

PART II: MAKING THE PLAN

F. Synthesize the previous information into a goal statement for your project.

G. Identify and briefly describe five (or more) objectives that will help you in reaching your goal for the project.

1.

2.

3.

4.

5.

H. For each objective, list the tasks (action items), time lines, and individuals responsible in reaching the objective. Name the objective.

Tasks	Beginning/ Ending Dates	Resources Needed to Reach Objectives	Individual Responsible

(Elhard & Lavalier, 2002)

I. List resources that are currently available and those that need to be obtained to reach the objectives.

Resources Currently Available	Resources Needed

J. If your plan includes volunteer work with an agency or organization, include

The name of the agency or organization and a brief explanation of how this agency is appropriate for your goals.

The arrangements you will need to make to complete the project.

The name and phone number of your contact person.

The hours and amount of time you will spend volunteering.

Special skills or knowledge that are required for the volunteer position.

PART III: JUSTIFICATION

K. Review your plan and make a final statement of justification for the experience you selected. Check to be sure it is realistic and likely to be attained. Is it feasible?

L. Describe why your project is important to both you and the community.

M. Provide concrete and specific data from each of the following to support your project.

    a. Brain research

    b. Preliminary data research

    c. Primary data research

    d. New project-specific data

N. Describe how you will evaluate your action plan. Include pre- and post-measurement plans to evaluate effectiveness in achieving the vision, goals, and objectives of your project.

Public Health Intervention Work Plan

Objective of the Intervention: _____

Assessment: _____

Equipment and Resources: _____

Place of Intervention: _____

Approximate Date of Intervention: _____

Administrative Permission: _____

Planning Tasks	Completed by Whom	Completed by When

Implementation Tasks	Completed by Whom	Completed by When

Evaluation Tasks	Completed by Whom	Completed by When

(Gast & Lounsberry, 2002)

Example of Integrating a Public Health Issue into Various Disciplines
Polio

Concepts by Discipline	Student Knowledge and Understanding
Language Arts	**Language Arts**
the emergence of mass media to disseminate information to the public	role playing
continuation of research methods	ethics/values surrounding the epidemic
	the poetry of "a man in an iron lung"
Social Studies	**Social Studies**
social and public nature of epidemics	specific strategies to combat an American epidemic
the impact of fear on American society in the 1950s	individual versus community responsibility
financing large scale health-related research	global inequities related to medical progress
government support and intervention	formation of NFIP/March of Dimes
rights of a handicapped individual	FDR and his public image
Science	**Science**
exploring different disease pathogens	comparison of viral and bacterial treatment
principles of scientific research	technology of vaccine development
high efficacy, low toxicity	double-blind study
ethics of research	placebo effect and control groups
Math	**Math**
controlled experimentation	experimental design
quantifying results of experimentation	simple random samples
the Salk vaccine trials' statistical significance	control groups
sampling	census versus sample
randomization	communicating numerical results—numerically, graphically, verbally
current drug trials/experiments (HIV/AIDS)	

(Grady, 2002)

Example of Integrating a Public Health Issue
into Various Disciplines
Polio *(continued)*

Curriculum Flow Chart	Student Activities/Assignments
Role of disease as selection pressure on civilizations Social, economic, political impact of epidemics throughout history (bubonic, typhus, smallpox)	Readings and activities from *Plagues and Peoples* by William McNeil
Research techniques—examine literary, scientific, and political information on polio	Media portrayal of victims, FDR advent of television
Characteristics of virus/vaccines	Readings from *Viral Structure* contrast of pathogens (cholera versus polio versus AIDS) Concepts of vaccines Treatment options

Historical look at the 1950s and polio	Readings
	    "In the Shadow of Polio" by Kathryn Black
	    "Fear of Polio in the 1950s" by Beth Sokol
	Group activity exploring five ethical dilemmas
	Integrating values with decisions through class discussions

Technological solutions
    case study of the Salk trials
    experimental design
    statistical methods of experimentation
    ethical issues of human experimentation
    mathematical modeling
	Calculations using Salk data
	Randomization activity using playing cards
	Problems and readings from
	    Statistics by David Moore
	Exponential, cubic growth
	Difference between census/sample

Comparison of polio treatments to current drug treatments	Results of AIDS drug trials Student-generated examples from current publications

Service Learning Reflection Activities

Reflection Assignments

The following reflection "prompts" encourage different types of critical thinking from students through various forms of expression:

- Draw a web showing what you already know about the topic of public health and what you would like to know. *(Recalling and organizing)*

- Write a letter to yourself before your service work begins. What do you predict that this experience will be like for you? *(Forecasting)*

- Create a flowchart to represent the steps involved in implementing your service learning project. *(Sequencing)*

- Write about a critical incident that happened in your service learning work where you didn't know what to do. How did you handle it? What would you change if this happened again? *(Problem-solving)*

- Draw a cartoon that teaches something important about the people you are serving. *(Synthesis and creative thinking)*

- If you were given the authority, how would you change this class or your service learning assignment? *(Evaluation)*

- Draw a diagram showing your before-and-after image of the people with whom you have been working. *(Compare and contrast)*

- Where and how might you use the knowledge that you have gained from your service learning project? *(Application)*

- What has your service work taught you about the type of career that you would like to have or not have? *(Application)*

Toole, J., & Toole, P. (1995). Reflection as a tool for turning service experiences into learning experiences. In C. W. Kinsley & K. McPherson (Eds.). *Enriching the Curriculum Through Service Learning* (p. 108). Alexandria, VA: Association for Supervision and Curriculum Development. Reprinted with permission.

Rubric for Evaluators

1. EVALUATION CRITERIA	EXPERT (5)	(4)	APPRENTICE (3)	(2)	NOVICE (1)
Visual display communicates effectively and creatively. SCORE: _____ COMMENTS:	The main focus of the project is immediately clear. The viewer's attention is grabbed and held by a varied array of colors, statistics, and images. A variety of methods are used to convey the message (including a theme statement, pictures, pamphlets or audiovisuals, and so forth). Text is free of misspellings and is grammatically correct.		The display communicates the project focus clearly. Visuals complement the main idea of the project. A viewer would have little problem understanding the message of the display. A variety of methods were used to convey the message, although a couple seemed undeveloped. Text is nearly free of grammatical and spelling errors.		The purpose of the project is not clear. Images and text are not complementary. The display does not catch or hold attention. Workmanship seems sloppy and unprofessional. Only one or two methods (text, charts, pictures, diagrams, quotes, and so forth) of relaying information. Errors in the text greatly detract from message of visual presentation.

2. EVALUATION CRITERIA	EXPERT (5)	(4)	APPRENTICE (3)	(2)	NOVICE (1)
The visual display and the oral presentation are presented in logical order. SCORE: _____ COMMENTS:	The community issue is explored in logical order (the current state of issue, nationally and locally, efforts being made locally, further needs, current solutions attempted by project, future projections). Materials are neat and attractively formatted. Oral presentation was obviously thoroughly planned and rehearsed.		Effort made to break visual and oral report into distinct parts. Diagrams, pictures, and charts may be effective in visual display, but not explained well in oral presentation. Oral presentation proceeds with only a few "bumps," a minimal amount of slang or mispronunciation.		No logical order in displays. Looks more like a collage. The oral presentation was unfocused and seemed as though participants were "winging it." Hard to follow to a logical conclusion.

(Elhard & Lavalier, 2002)

Rubric for Evaluators *(continued)*

3. EVALUATION CRITERIA	EXPERT (5)	(4)	APPRENTICE (3)	(2)	NOVICE (1)
Knowledge of subject. SCORE: _____ COMMENTS:	The student seems well-versed on recent research in subject area. Quantitative and qualitative evidence is supplied. A few prominent researchers are cited in the display and presentation. Local experts were also consulted through interviews or authentic interaction. Overall, the presenter had a rich, deep knowledge and understanding of the complexity of this issue. At least 10 sources cited.		The student shows evidence of research. References to research are made but may not indicate a sophisticated knowledge of what it means. Sources cited may show gaps (e.g., few, if any, interviews of local experts). Research may show signs of being somewhat outdated. Able to explain all portions of the poster in a clear, knowledgeable manner.		The student has a general knowledge of the topic but used many unsupported statements. Little if any research mentioned. Talked as though the subject was fairly simple and uncomplicated. Little evidence of a change in thinking produced by examination of the topic. Bibliography shows a great imbalance toward national or local sources.

4. EVALUATION CRITERIA	EXPERT (5)	(4)	APPRENTICE (3)	(2)	NOVICE (1)
Questions are answered respectfully and professionally. SCORE: _____ COMMENTS:	All questions are treated as good questions. Students are capable of responding directly to what is asked in most cases. Examples of experience and relevant research are used in their responses. Encouraged the audience to ask questions.		Most questions are given serious consideration. Students give relevant answers, although they may stray from original intent. General theories or examples are used. Accepted questions but did not try to elicit them.		Answers are short and sound "off the cuff." Sarcasm or lack of tact may be evident. No eye contact used. One student monopolizes the talking. Discouraged audience from asking questions.

Rubric for Evaluators *(continued)*

5. EVALUATION CRITERIA	EXPERT (5)	(4)	APPRENTICE (3)	(2)	NOVICE (1)
Written product (e.g., handout, book, pamphlet) communicates a strong, clear message of why this issue is important. SCORE: ____ COMMENTS:	Handout could stand alone as an effective communication of the issue. Awareness and concern are raised in the reading. Solution or recommendations are offered. An appropriate amount of data and statistics is used. Message is memorable. Text is grammatically correct and free of misspellings.		Handout supplements the presentation. Data are relevant and informative. May not make the case for a community initiative to improve the issue of concern. Seems consistent with oral presentation. Text is clear and easy to read.		Handout provides a sketch of the issue. The text has no real order and seems more like a fact sheet. Little attempt to persuade the audience to take action. The reading material is messy. No graphics or variation in the text. Poor grammar and misspellings may be present.

6. EVALUATION CRITERIA	EXPERT (5)	(4)	APPRENTICE (3)	(2)	NOVICE (1)
Personal appearance and communication skills. SCORE: ____ COMMENTS:	Looked the part of a professional. Acted in a mature, adult manner. Presenters were courteous to each other and to their audience. Presenters were enthusiastic in voice and action. Good eye contact and voice inflection.		Appearance is adequate but may have something that distracts from their message. May be inconsistent in their treatment of people. May be lacking in some key speaking area: eye contact, pronunciation, confidence, voice inflection, enthusiasm, and so forth.		Appearance was unkempt and unprofessional. Distracted others or were easily distracted themselves. Used slang or grunts to communicate (unless demonstrating speech development in infants). Speech hard to understand or monotone.

Rubric for Evaluators *(continued)*

7. EVALUATION CRITERIA	EXPERT (5)	(4)	APPRENTICE (3)	(2)	NOVICE (1)
Future-oriented attitude. SCORE: _____ COMMENTS:	This project has strong potential to become a long-term initiative. Dreams, hopes, or plans for future actions are explicitly stated. Prevention of problem behavior, unhealthy habits, or antisocial attitudes seems to be the aim. Persuasive in demonstrating that this project and related follow-up endeavors will make a difference in our community.		This project, with some revision or restructuring, could be a viable project for future groups in community issues class. They express a hope for someone to carry on their work next year. Prevention is stressed. The desire to improve the community is an implicit message they conveyed.		The project seems as if it would be hard to replicate or build from. No mention of the future. Seems resigned to the "fact" that little can be done to improve this issue. The presenters seem mostly self-oriented and don't demonstrate a concern for the greater community.

Urban Public Health
School of Health Sciences
Phone (212) 481-5111
Fax (212) 481-5260

HUNTER COLLEGE
OF THE CITY UNIVERSITY OF NEW YORK

COLLEGE EXPLORATORY PROGRAM IN PUBLIC HEALTH
CLOSING ACTIVITY

Dear Taft High School Student:

Remember the T-shirt activity at our first meeting when you imagined what you would be doing ten years from now and then drew pictures on the T-shirt of your goals?

Well, now we'd like you to think about where you will be and what you will be doing in one year and three years from now. Then on separate pieces of paper, write a letter to yourself as if it were one year and three years later. Describe what you are doing, where you are living, whether you are in school, or working, or whatever! Be as imaginative as you'd like, but base your writing on some real goals that you've set for yourself.

Then, seal each letter in separate envelopes and address them to yourself at your home address (if you or your family members expect to still be living there in 2003 and 2005) or to the address of another family member or relative who you expect will remain at that location for the next three years.

Turn in your sealed letters to us. We will then mail them to you next year (and in three years) along with a letter from us asking what you are actually doing. Open your letter from yourself and see how close you came to "predicting" your future. Did you imagine right? Or are you doing something completely different? Are you surprised by what you are doing? Are you pleased? How do you feel about things in your life right now?

At that time, we'll send you a self-addressed envelope, too, so you can share with us what's going on in your life and whether things are going as you expected or if they are completely different.

We're sure that whatever you will be doing, you'll be doing it well and succeeding in your efforts! It's been a wonderful experience having you in this program and we wish all good things for you in the future.

Very best of luck, stay well, and keep at it!

Sincerely,

Gerry Zuzze, MPH   Lynn Roberts, PhD
Evaluator   Principal Investigator

Education, Action and Research for a Healthier New York
Brookdale Health Science Center   425 East 25th Street New York NY 10010

(Roberts, Cordero & Pichardo, 2002)

Lead Smarts Outreach Outcomes

During the 2002/2003 Academic Year

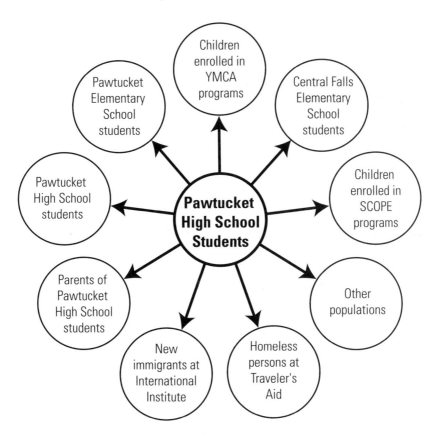

(Wooler & Herman, 2002)

Resources
for Educators

Bibliography

Allen, L., & Lunsford, B. (1995). *How to form networks for school renewal.* Alexandria, VA: Association for Supervision and Curriculum Development.

Allen, R. (2003, March). The democratic aims of service learning. *Educational Leadership, 60*(6), 51–54.

Battistich, V., & Hom, A. (1997, December). The relationship between students' sense of their school as a community and their involvement in problem behaviors. *American Journal of Public Health, 87*(12), 1997–2001.

Billig, S. H. (2000, May). Research on K-12 school-based service learning: The evidence builds. *Phi Delta Kappan, 81*(9), 658–664.

Camp, W. G. (2001, May/June). Participation in student activities and achievement: A covariance structural analysis. *Journal of Educational Research, 83*(5), 272–278.

Center for Mental Health in Schools. (2002, October). Weaving school-community resources together. In *A center concept paper and accompanying resource aids: Rethinking student support to enable students to learn and schools to teach.* Los Angeles: Author.

Checkley, K., & Rasmussen, K. (1997, Summer). Problem-based learning. *Curriculum Update,* pp. 1–8.

Council of Chief State Schools Officers. (1998). [Issue brief.] *Ensuring student success through collaboration: State education agency support for school-community collaboration in the mid-Atlantic states.* Washington, DC: Author.

Delisle, R. (1997). *How to use problem-based learning in the classroom.* Alexandria, VA: Association for Supervision and Curriculum Development.

Edmondson, J., Thorson, G., & Fluegel, D. (2000, April). Big school change in a small town. *Educational Leadership, 57*(7), 51–53.

Epstein, J. L. (1995, May). School/family/community partnerships: Caring for the children we share. *Phi Delta Kappan,* pp. 701–713.

Ernst, D., & Amis, B. (1999). Service learning: A growing movement. *ASCD Infobrief, 19,* 1–8.

Fullan, M. (2002, May). The change leader. *Educational Leadership, 59*(8), 16–20.

Glickman, C. D. (2003). Going public: The imperative of public education in the twenty-first century. In C. D. Glickman, *Holding sacred ground: Essays on leadership, courage, and endurance in our schools* (pp. 301–311). San Francisco: Jossey-Bass.

Glickman, C. D. (2003). Leadership for navigating great American schools. In C. D. Glickman, Holding sacred ground: Essays on leadership, courage, and endurance in our schools (pp. 11–25). San Francisco: Jossey-Bass.

Green, L. W., & Kreuter, M. W. (1991). *Health promotion planning: An educational and environmental approach* (3rd ed.). Mountain View, CA: Mayfield Publishing Company.

Haber, D., & Blaber, C. (1995). Health education: A foundation for learning. In A. A. Glatthorn (Ed.), *Content of the curriculum* (2nd ed.) (Chapter 5). Alexandria, VA: Association for Supervision and Curriculum Development.

Hawkins, D. J., & Catalano, R. F. (1990). Broadening the vision of education: Schools as health promoting environments. *American School Association Journal of School Health, 60*(4), 178–186.

Jacobs, H. H. (1991, October). Planning for curriculum integration. *Educational Leadership, 49*(2), 27–28.

Kinsley, C. W., & McPherson, K. (Eds.). (1995). *Enriching the curriculum through service learning.* Alexandria, VA: Association for Supervision and Curriculum Development.

Kysilka, M. L. (1998, Summer). Understanding integrated curriculum. *The Curriculum Journal, 9*(2),198–209.

Mahoney, J. L. (2000, March/April). School extracurricular activity participation as a moderator in the development of antisocial patterns. *Child Development, 71*(2), 502–516.

Marzano, R. J., Pickering, D., & McTighe, J. (1993). *Assessing student outcomes: Performance assessment using the dimensions of learning model.* Alexandria, VA: Association for Supervision and Curriculum Development.

National Association of State Boards of Education. (2003). *How schools work and how to work with schools.* Alexandria, VA: Author.

Negroni, P. J. (1995). Vision for the 21st century: Seamless relationship between school and community (Chapter 13). In C. W. Kinsley & K. McPherson (Eds.), *Enriching the curriculum through service learning* (Chapter 13). Alexandria, VA: Association for Supervision and Curriculum Development.

Novick, B. (2002). *Building learning communities with character: How to integrate academic, social, and emotional learning.* Alexandria, VA: Association for Supervision and Curriculum Development.

O'Brien, E., & Rollefson, M. (1995, June). *Extracurricular participation and student engagement* [Report NCES 95-741]. Washington, DC: U.S. Department of Education, Office of Educational Research and Improvement.

Rhem, J. (1998). Problem-based learning: An introduction. *The National Teaching & Learning Forum, 8*(1), 4–7.

Sedo, J., & Hindle, D. R. (2000, Spring). Building the caring school community. *Education Canada, 40*(1), 40–44.

Stone, C. R. (1995, May). School/community collaboration: comparing three initiatives. *Phi Delta Kappan,* pp. 794–804.

Stoto, M. A., Abel, C. and Dievler, A. (Eds.). (1996). *Healthy communities: New partnerships for the future of public health.* Washington, DC: National Academy Press.

Taylor, L., & Adelman, H. S. (2000, June). Connecting schools, families, and communities. *Professional School Counseling, 3*(5), 298–308.

Torp, L., & Sage, S. (2002). *Problems as possibilities: Problem-based learning for K-16 education* (2nd ed.). Alexandria, VA: Association for Supervision and Curriculum Development.

Welch, M., & Sheridan, S. M. (1995). *Educational partnerships: Serving students at risk.* Fort Worth, TX: Harcourt Brace.

Westbrook, J. M., & Albert, S. V. (2002). *Creating the capacity for change.* Alexandria, VA: Association for Supervision and Curriculum Development.

Witmer, J. T., & Anderson, C. S. (1994). *How to establish a high school service learning program.* Alexandria, VA: Association for Supervision and Curriculum Development.

Internet Resources

1. **Public health information**
   - The Division of Adolescent and School Health (DASH), a part of the Centers for Disease Control and Prevention, identifies and monitors highest-priority risks, applies research, implements national programs to prevent these risks, and evaluates the programs. http://www.cdc.gov/nccdphp/dash
   - The Centers for Disease Control and Prevention conducted the School Health Policies and Programs Study in 1994 and 2000. Along with a description of the results of this study, the Web site contains useful information on state and district health policies and practices. http://www.cdc.gov/shpps
   - Association of Schools of Public Health has general information on public health, reports on public health, job listings, and Schools of Public Health. http://www.asph.org
   - Office of Minority Health Resource Center was established by the U.S. Department of Health and Human Services to serve as a national resource and referral service on minority health issues. http://www.omhrc.gov/omhrc
   - EthnoMed, a Web site sponsored by the University of Washington's Harborview Medical Center, includes information about the health care practices and expectations of different cultures. http://www.ethnomed.org
   - ASCD's Health in Education Initiative features articles exploring the current state of public health in the United States and describes its program to stimulate partnerships between schools and public health organizations to increase students' knowledge of issues, methods, and careers in public health. http://www.ascd.org/health_in_education/index.html

2. **Classroom resources: standards, data, and materials**
   - The National Standards for School Health Education, released in 1995 by the U.S. Department of Education, identifies standards students must achieve to become health literate. http://www.ed.gov/databases/ERIC_Digests/ed387483.html

- The Youth Risk Behavior Surveillance System (YRBSS), a program of the Centers for Disease Control and Prevention, monitors health-risk behaviors that significantly contribute to the leading causes of death, disability, and social problems among youth and adults in this country. CDC-DASH conducts a survey every two years to gather data on high school students. http://www.cdc.gov/nccdphp/dash/yrbs

- *America's Children: Key National Indicators of Well-Being* is an annual report on the status of the nation's children from the Federal Interagency Forum on Child and Family Statistics. http://childstats.gov/americaschildren

- The State Collaborative on Assessment and Student Standards created the Health Education Assessment Project to identify and develop measures of assessment in health education. http://www.ccsso.org/projects/SCASS/Projects/Health_Education_Assessment_Project

- Kids Count, a project of the Annie E. Casey Foundation, is a state-by-state effort to track the status and well-being of children across the country. The Web site includes reports and data on specific states. http://www.aecf.org/kidscount

- The National Center for Health Statistics, a division of the Centers for Disease Control and Prevention, has lots of data. A report called *Health, United States, 2000 With Adolescent Chartbook* has specific information on the status of adolescent health. http://www.cdc.gov/nchs/data/hus/hus00.pdf

- The National Health Information Center has a database of more than 1,800 organizations and government offices that provide information upon request. http://www.health.gov/nhic/AlphaKeyword.htm

- PBS TeacherSource: Health & Fitness has articles and other resources for educators. http://www.pbs.org/teachersource/health.htm

- National Institute of Environmental Health Sciences has free resources for teachers interested in environmental health issues. http://www.niehs.nih.gov/external/teacher.htm

- HealthTeacher provides information on health literacy and curriculum tools for health education; it guides teachers through a step-by-step process to develop lesson plans. There is a subscription fee. http://www.healthteacher.com

- American School Health Association (ASHA) has conferences and publications to promote the health of youth. ASHA is a membership organization, but its publications are available for purchase by non-members. http://www.ashaweb.org

3. **Service learning**

- Learning In Deed is an initiative of the Kellogg Foundation to inform and involve people in service learning. The Web site provides resources and tools for educators, students, and policymakers. http://learningindeed.org

- National Service-Learning Clearinghouse has information about service learning, trends, conferences and events, news updates, and funding sources. It also provides resources, tools, and technical assistance. http://www.servicelearning.org

- National Youth Leadership Council's mission is to involve young people in building vital, just communities through service learning. The organization has a strong advocacy component, resources, and articles. http://www.nylc.org

- Learn and Serve America is a program of the Corporation for National Service that provides opportunities throughout the country for young people to get involved in serving their communities. http://www.learnandserve.org

- Compact for Learning and Citizenship, founded by the Education Commission of the States, is a nationwide coalition that gathers and disseminates information, provides training and technical assistance, builds partnerships and networks, and serves as a national voice for creating high-quality service learning opportunities for all students. http://www.ecs.org/ecsmain.asp?page=/search/default.asp

4. **Funding**

- The Centers for Disease Control and Prevention's Division of Adolescent and School Health maintains a continually updated database of federal, foundation, and state funding opportunities for schools interested in developing or improving their school health programs. http://www.cdc.gov/nccdphp/dash/funding/index.htm

- Schools can find out how health program funds are being used in their state by visiting the National Conference of State Legislatures Web site. http://www.ncsl.org/programs/health/pp/schlfund.htm

5. **Community partnerships**

- The Community Toolbox: Bringing Solutions to Light is a free, Internet-based service that assists people in addressing community health and development issues in *their* community. The Toolbox includes materials for building healthy communities, including step-by-step guidelines, real-life examples, checklists, and training materials. http://ctb.ku.edu

Advisory Committee
Health in Education Initiative

Charles Deutsch
Director
Partnership for Children's Health
Harvard School of Public Health

Deborah Haber
Educational Development Center
Project Director, Center for School Health

Gerald Lewis
Principal, J.C. Harmon High School
Kansas City, Kansas

Charles Patterson
Superintendent of Schools
Killeen, Texas, Independent School District

William T. Small
Dean Emeritus, School of Public Health
University of North Carolina, Chapel Hill

Jane Tustin
Coordinator, Health Services
Lubbock, Texas, Independent School District

About the Author

Jenny Smith has researched, written, and worked on the production of award-winning public affairs documentaries for PBS television. She helped produce several shows that covered education, including *Surviving the Bottom Line*, winner of the 1999 CINE Golden Eagle award. She researched and wrote about education reform efforts in high-poverty urban areas nationwide for a Ford Foundation Research & Development grant. Smith is the author of *Exemplary Assessment: Measurement That's Useful*, an ASCD PD Online.

Smith holds a master's degree in the field of psychology and has worked with adults and children in mental health clinic and school settings. She is also the co-author of the children's book *A Spark in the Dark*, which is featured on the award-winning CD and cassette titled *A Planet with One Mind*.